Home Treatment With the Cell-salts

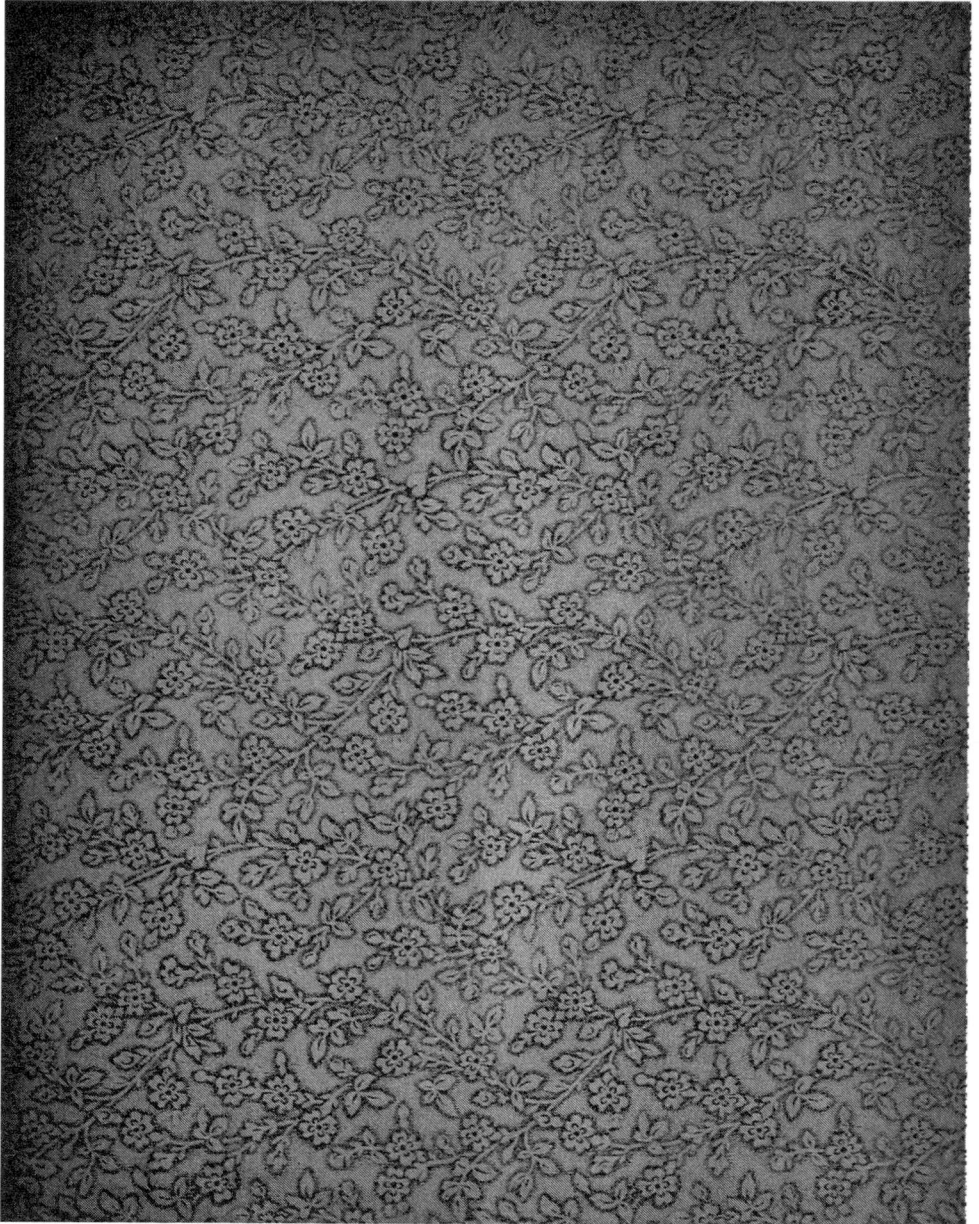

S. H. PLATT.

HOME TREATMENT

WITH THE

CELL-SALTS.

BY

S. H. PLATT,

AUTHOR OF——

"PRINCELY MANHOOD,"
"QUEENLY WOMANHOOD,"
"OUR SPECIAL ADVISER,"
"THE SECRETS OF HEALTH,"
"THE POWER OF GRACE,"
"THE PHILOSOPHY OF CHRISTIAN HOLINESS,"
"THE MAN OF LIKE PASSIONS,"
"THE WONDROUS NAME,"

AND WRITER OF

"TALKS WITH OUR DOCTOR,"
AND
"OUR HEALTH ADVISER."

PUBLISHED BY

E. F. BARNES, SOUTHERN PINES, N. C.

1897.

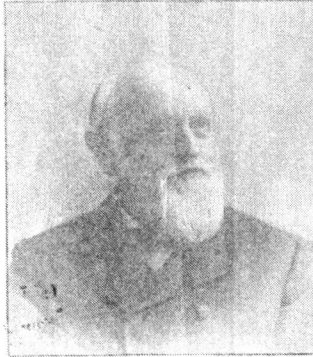

A. H. HAYT

HOME TREATMENT

WITH THE

CELL-SALTS,

BY

S. H. PLATT.

AUTHOR OF

"PRINCELY MANHOOD,"
"QUEENLY WOMANHOOD,"
"OUR SPECIAL ADVISER,"
"THE SECRETS OF HEALTH,"
"THE POWER OF GRACE,"
"THE PHILOSOPHY OF CHRISTIAN HOLINESS,"
"THE MAN OF LIKE PASSIONS,"
"THE WONDROUS NAME,"

AND WRITER OF

"TALKS WITH OUR DOCTOR,"
AND
"OUR HEALTH ADVISER."

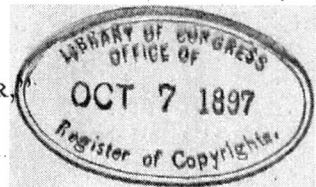

PUBLISHED BY

E. F. BARNES, SOUTHERN PINES, N. C.

1897.

CAPITAL PRINTING CO., RALEIGH, N. C.

OUTLINE PLAN.

CHAPTER ONE.

THE NEED OF A SAFE AND EFFICIENT HOME TREATMENT.

Shown by the fact that *some* home practice is almost always used before calling a physician; that very many are obliged to rely upon one *all through* sickness; that as constructed, there is serious danger that the nature of the disease will be mistaken; that there is great danger that the prescribed remedies will be misapplied; that eminent physicians confess the harmfulness of drug-dosing, even by their own hands; that an over-dose is detrimental and may be fatal; the Biochemic system only, prevents disaster in such circumstances.

CHAPTER TWO.

THE EFFICIENCY OF THE CELL-SALTS.

Demonstrated by the citation of hundreds of cases of people cured by them, as attested in the clinical reports of physicians to physicians (i. e. to medical societies and medical journals, not designed for the eye of the people), therefore absolutely reliable.

CHAPTER THREE.

THE BIOCHEMIC SYSTEM OF CURE FULLY EXPLAINED.

What disease is; what the Cell-Salts are; their properties and functions; *how* they cure disease.

CHAPTER FOUR.

THE INDICATIONS OR SYMPTOMS THAT CALL FOR THE USE OF EACH CELL-SALT.

All known symptoms of all diseases, so far as they relate to Biochemic remedies, are here classified, not by the names of diseases, for they are of no value, but by the functions and organs, e. g., digestion, thought, heat-production, etc., so that all confusion is avoided.

CHAPTER FIVE.

NATURE'S CO-OPERATIVE CURATIVES.

Diet, baths, exercise, sleep, rest, recreation, etc.

CHAPTER SIX.

THE CO-OPERATIVE CURATIVES OF SCIENCE.

When diseases become bacterial the Cell-Salts need to be reinforced by germicides   Which germicides are safe and efficient, and how to employ them.

CHAPTER SEVEN.

THE INDEPENDENT AND THE CO-OPERATIVE CURATIVES OF CHRISTIAN FAITH

INTRODUCTION.

The most natural as well as the most philosophical arrangement of a book for the home treatment of diseases is neither by the ordinary medical classifications, nor by regions as head, stomach, pelvis, etc., but by FUNCTIONS, for of what use is a head if it cannot think, or of a heart if it does not beat, or of a stomach if it cannot digest?

Therefore this book is a treatment of diseases by the functional derangements that they exhibit, and by which their presence is known.

If this new method seem inconvenient at first sight to the reader, he has but to glance at the *Outline Plan* next to the title page to see its comprehensiveness, symmetry and utility.·

And if one is at a loss to know under what function some symptom may be found, a moment's examination of the Index-Glossary will disclose it.

Biochemistry discards as unphilosophical and unscientific the names and classifications of diseases as they are found in the medical text books.

Why not then, have an arrangement of its own, based upon its own cardinal principles, and in harmony with its own use of remedies?

The important point to be fixed in the mind of the reader is that *names of diseases signify nothing*.

The functional disturbance is what is to be studied, and to THAT, not to a name, the remedies are to be fitted.

Other books lay down treatment for certain diseases which are to be distinguished by a few detailed symptoms, but as a matter of fact, the similarity between the symptoms is so close, and the frequency of other symptoms that

are not named is so great, that laymen are at their wit's
end to *know* just what disease to treat, and there is a period
in the onset of febrile diseases when not a physician on
earth can tell with certainty whether he has one disease or
another to combat.

All this perplexity is avoided by our method.

A fever is a functional disturbance of the circulation,
and should be treated as that purely and simply, without
regard to anything that may follow.

Of course this cannot be safely done in the use of drug-
poisons. Prof. Alonzo Clark says, "All our curative
agents (so-called) are poisons, and as a consequence every
dose diminishes the patient's vitality." But our remedies
are RECONSTRUCTIVE always, therefore are always *safe;* a
consideration of immense moment in placing curatives in
the hands of the people.   •

Medicines have been defined by Dr. C. Wesselhoeft in
a lecture before the advanced students of Harvard Medical School as "substances which if consumed by a well
person will make that well person sick."

According to this accepted definition the Biochemic
Salts are not medicines.

Very well; why employ medicines when remedies (re-
constructives) are efficient to cure? The use of this book
will demonstrate the superiority of remedies over medicines, and the utter uselessness of the latter, except as germicides in appropriate cases, as explained in Chapter VI.

Those who recognize diseases only by their names find
it hard to understand how one remedy can be appropriate
for many and dissimilar diseases.

But when they come to see that the same condition un-
derlies these diseases and that the true philosophy of cure
consists in *changing* that *condition*, then the beautiful sim-

plicity of the system explained in these pages becomes apparent.

Why should two thousand medicines be needed to correct the wrong conditions of the *few* elements out of which man is made?

Nature is severely simple in her methods ; man is ostentatiously complex in his.

The author is indebted to the following named Biochemic Works for the information that is gathered into this book, and to its publisher for much valuable assistance.

Abridged Therapeutics, founded upon Histology and Cellular Pathology, by Dr. W. H. Schuessler, translated by T. O. Connor, M. D. ; also a translation by Dr. M. Docetti Walker.

The Twelve Tissue Remedies, by Doctors Boericke and Dewey.

The Biochemic System of Medicine, by Dr. Geo. W. Carey.

The Tissue Remedies, by Dr. S. F. Shannon.

A Regional and Comparative Materia Medica, by Drs. John Gilmore Malcolm and Oscar Burnham Moss.

If the sum of human sufferings may be diminished by the aid of this effort, the author will feel profoundly grateful that he has been permitted under a beneficent Providence to have some share in the kindly work.

June 3, 1897.   S. H. PLATT.

CHAPTER I.

THE NEED OF A SAFE AND EFFICIENT HOME TREATMENT.

The general need of a safe and reliable system of home practice is apparent from these considerations, viz.:

1. The fact that some home practice is almost always resorted to before calling a physician. It may be to avoid the expense of the physician's services, or the immediate relief of pain, or from the general feeling that "something ought to be done," but for some reason home efforts *are* and will be made. Therefore it is important that they be rightly directed.

2. The limited resources of families, or their distance from physicians in whom they have confidence, necessitates reliance upon home practice *all through* many sicknesses, to the exclusion of all other helps. It may be a hard necessity, but very many, especially in thinly-settled regions, must combine in one person the office of parent, nurse and physician all through the weary, anxious hours of lingering sickness even to the end, be that end life or death. That the chances for life will be greatly augmented by a safe and efficient home practice none who believe in the law of cause and effect can doubt.

And common humanity strongly insists that if the end must be bereavement, the sufferers have the best aid that a reliable home system of practice can give, so that they may be solaced as others who employ physicians are, by the reflection, "all was done that could be" for recovery.

3. Home practice as ordinarily found is fraught with the serious danger of the great probability that the nature of the disease may be mistaken, i. e., wrong diagnosis made.

Medical books describe hundreds of diseases, each with its own peculiar symptoms, yet many resembling each other so closely that ordinary physicians are often unable to di-criminate between them, and a skillful diagnostican (one who diagnoses or detects disease) is among the rarest of medical experts. That the common people should mistake the disease is therefore the most probable of all probable things, and if the error does occur no one can tell the mischief that may result. Hence it is a common experience of physicians to find diseases seriously aggravated by the mistakes of home efforts to relieve. It is therefore of great consequence that those efforts, if they cannot be free from a mistaken direc.ion, may at least escape the the baneful results of injurious medication.

4. Home practice as ordinarily prescribed in books of home treatment is attended with the great probability that the remedies will be misapplied.

If they are allophatic or eclectic, some in most frequent use are deadly poisons ; many are in their nature deleterious, and nearly all are over-dosed. The narcotics, opiates, sedatives, stimulants, etc., most generally prescribed would amaze an intelligent observer were he not so accustomed to the sight. But familiarity with them does not change the nature of opium, chloral, nux vomica, digitalis or the bromides.

Physicians deplore the uncertainty which attends the administration of the most deadly drugs arising from the variations in the proportions of their active principles in different preparations, e. g., opium may contain eight or sixteen per cent of morphine to the grain, i. e., one dose may be one dose, or it may be two. Belladonna contains atropine varying from 0.25 per cent to 0.75 per cent.

Other drugs vary still more widely, yet the books dose

the drug at a fixed quantity, and physicians prescribe them accordingly.

But the " accidents " are attributed to other causes, and so the death-dealing work goes on.

Is it likely to be any less when the same drugs are employed in home prescriptions?

If the medicines are homeopathic, the poisons are prescribed more frequently than the harmless agents, and if they have any efficiency to heal when wisely used, they are equally efficient to injure if unwisely employed. And that they must be unwisely employed is a necessity arising from the complexity of the system itself. Says Dr. H. A. Anderson, " When we give four thousand symptoms with aggravations for nearly every hour of the day to a single drug, it is a confusion to the student and a stumbling-block to the experienced prescriber."

The writer has personally examined the case of a homeopathic physician, consisting of sixteen hundred vials, each containing a remedy different in nature or potency from all the others. Now a system that requires sixteen hundred remedies to treat some thousands of " indications " is certain to have its remedies misapplied by laymen or physicians either, unless they are experts.

It is absurd to say that " if they do no good they will do no harm." If they have no potency, the system is a fraud, and they who recommend it are abettors of fraud. If they have potency, it is for good or ill according as it is wisely or unwisely applied, and the point that I insist upon is, that unwise application is unavoidable in the case of all but experts. Therefore remedies that are harmless are a prime necessity for home treatment of disease.

To add to the certainty that serious results will be likely to occur in the home use of drug medicines is the fact that they are so generally adulterated that no certainty can be had of securing from the ordinary druggist the medicine that is ordered. As an illustration, the New York Pharmaceutical Association reports that " seven samples of nitrous ether varied so greatly that a pint of one only equaled a teaspoonful of another." A manufacturing pharmacist sent fifty prescriptions precisely alike to fifty drug stores. It called for one article that all drug stores are supposed to keep in stock. Analyses showed that only about three of the fifty were correctly put up, and a large proportion of them did not contain a particle of the test medicine.

They who use drugs in home prescriptions are certain to deal with most uncertain agents.

5. No person who has read the confessions of noted physicians relative to the uncertainty and harmfulness of the ordinary drug treatment of disease can doubt that a better system of cure is one of the most pressing needs of life.

For example, Dr. Sidney Ringer, the greatest English authority on the action of drugs, says: " The sustained administration of alkalies and their carbonates renders the blood *poorer in solids and in red corpuscles*, and impairs the nutrition of the body."

So Dr. Wood, endorsed by Dr. W. L. Stowell, American Medical Bulletin, says: " Present therapeutics is a mixture of science and empiricism." Also Dr. J. J. M. Goss, in Medical Brief, says: " Medicine lacks much of being a fixed science."

" Ninety-nine out of every hundred medical facts are medical lies ; and medical doctrines are for the most part, stark, staring nonsense."—*Professor Gregory, Edinburgh.*

" Medicine is a barbarous jargon, and has destroyed

more lives than war, pestilence and famine combined."—
John Mason Good, M. D., F. R. S.

"Thousands are annually slaughtered in the quiet sick
room. Governments should banish medical men and pro-
scribe their blundering art."—*Dr. Titus, Counselor of the
Court at Dresden.*

"The stolid bigotry which will not be enlightened and ·
will not investigate is responsible for many millions of
deaths. The gigantic errors of medical men need vigorous
criticism by those who are not afraid to speak.—*Dr. Bu-
chanan.*

"Drugs do not act in the beneficial way they are supposed to do ; according to my reading they are so many
poisons, and I am supported by medical books, which
speak of the toxic (poisonous) effects of drugs. Many
cases are made worse, or recovery is protracted by the use
of drugs, whilst some are even killed or their death hastened by the drugs themselves."—*Dr. Allinson, London.*

"Medicine is a great humbug.· I know it is called science. Science, indeed! it is nothing like science. Doctors are merely empirics when they are not charlatans."—
M. Magendie, the celebrated French physiologist.

"All medicines which enter the circulation poison the
blood in the same manner as do the poisons that produce
the disease. Drugs do not cure disease. Digitalis has
hurried thousands to the grave. Prussic acid was once
extensively used in the treatment of consumption, both in
Europe and America, but its reputation is lost. Thousands of patients were treated with it, but not a case was
benefited. On the contrary, hundreds were hurried to the
grave."—*The venerable Prof. Jos. M. Smith, M. D.*

"All our curative agents (so-called) are poisons, and as

a consequence every dose diminishes the patient's vitality."—*Prof. Alonzo Clark, M. D.*

"The medical practice of our day is, at the best, a most uncertain and unsatisfactory system; it has neither philosophy nor common sense to commend it to confidence." —*Prof. Evans, Fellow of the Royal College, London, England.*

"Our actual information or knowledge of disease does not increase in proportion to our experimental practice. Every dose of medicine given is a blind experiment upon the vitality of the patient."—*Dr. Bostick, author of History of Medicine.*

"Dissections daily convince us of our ignorance of disease and cause us to blush at our prescriptions. What mischiefs have we not done under the belief of false facts and false theories? We have assisted in multiplying disease; we have done more; we have increased their fatality."—*Benjamin Rush, M. D., Philadelphia.*

"The drugs which are administered for the cure of scarlet fever and measles kill far more than the diseases do. Instead of investigating for themselves, medical authorities have copied the errors of predecessors, and have thus retarded progress and perpetuated errors."—*Prof. B. F. Barker, M. D.*

6. An over-dose of the remedies of the systems to which the above citations refer produce disturbance of the functions in proportion to the dose.

Official reports from seven European hospitals show under homeopathic treatment a mortality of 4.22 per cent.

Official reports from five European hospitals under allopathic care give a death rate of 12.61 per cent., thus showing the beneficent effects of the least medication as compared with the freer use of drugs, even in the hands of skilled physicians.

The cell-salt remedies if over-dosed or misapplied are simply not appropriated by the absorbents and are carried as waste matter out of the body with no functional disturbance. Therefore they are perfectly safe.

No person who is familiar with the figures showing the enormous sale of patent and proprietary medicines can doubt that the *people* have taken the work of curing their countless ailments into *their own hands*. They buy and take *blindly* because they do not know what better thing to do.

Home treatment doctor books representing all the leading "pathies" have been sold broadcast, yet the people feel that the RIGHT SYSTEM has not come to them yet.

Fortunately, this can be said no longer. The Biochemic System is the most safe, scientific and satisfactory theory and practice of cure that the world has ever seen.

It was not elaborated for the use of the people, and for thirty years has been kept from them.

This book is the first systematic effort that has ever been made in the English language to adapt the system to the comprehension, and adjust the treatment to the use of those who know nothing of the sciences that are supposed to be a necessary part of a medical education.

Can it be done? Unquestionably it can, for among the author's own patrons it HAS BEEN successfully employed in very many instances. And why not? No acquaintance with anatomy, physiology, chemistry, materia medica (medical substances) nor therapeutics (to cure by remedies) is necessary in the home use of the cell-salts.

Names of diseases are entirely ignored, and *conditions* only are considered.

These conditions are not some hidden, mysterious things that only a doctor can discriminate, but such as the color of the coat of the tongue, the color and consistency of expectoration or of a discharge, the kind of pain, i. e., shifting or steady, shooting or grinding, etc. Surely these matters ANY PERSON OF ORDINARY INTELLIGENCE can determine positively, and with that knowledge he has only to ask this book what salt to use in such conditions, and it answers with a certainty that is as unfailing as human judgment can make it, and is as refreshing as it is sure when compared with the timid, hesitating uncertainty that most people feel in the use of the home doctor books and drug medicines of the past.

This great fact only has but to be stated to show the absolute superiority of this practice over all others, and the necessity for it, because it is thus superior.

THE PEOPLE OUGHT TO HAVE THE BEST.

CHAPTER II.

THE EFFICIENCY OF THE CELL-SALTS.

There are two methods of determining this question.

The first is the one pursued by patent medicine manufacturers, viz., the collection of *testimonials* from those who as patients have used the nostrums and certify to their value.

The objections to this class of evidence are:

1. The very great liability to *mistake* on the part of those unfamiliar with diseases, and their consequent false report of their real condition.

2. The nearly universal tendency of the human mind to make reports as startling as possible—thus leading to exaggeration.

3. The fact that such testimonies are often *influenced*, sometimes bought outright, and sometimes *transferred* from one article to another.

4. The fact that no nostrum is ever found so poor in virtue that large numbers of testimonials are not offered in its favor.

This item alone should cause the acceptance of such evidence to be considered as a very weak foundation on which to rest the use of compounds affecting human life.

The other method of reaching the truth as to the efficiency of the Cell-Salts is:

To collect testimonials from PHYSICIANS who have prescribed them, and who certify their value in specific conditions to their fellow physicians, whose knowledge of the import of those conditions furnishes a safeguard against undue exaggeration, and who, by the very circumstances in which the testimony is given, can neither be influenced nor bought. '

Such evidence from professional men is the strongest that can possibly be adduced outside of a court of justice.

, Such is the testimony that is here cited.

These reports are also of peculiar value as detailed *examples* of the actual use of the remedies in every-day practice, thus furnishing to the intelligent layman hints of the wise selection for the conditions named.

Surely the same remedies for the same conditions can be no less efficient if dealt out by unprofessional hands.

It will be observed that in some cases potences other than the 6x are employed.

This is well enough for physicians, but as Schuessler advised, the 6x should be the standard, only to be departed from when that obviously fails, not because wrongly selected, but because the system of the patient is incompetent to assimilate it. In most of these cases cited herein there is no evidence that 6x would not have done as well as the potency actually employed.

The life-long habits of drug dosing have created a timidity in the use of remedies unless specifically prescribed by professional authority on the part of many who rely upon their physicians only, but such need not fear to follow these prescriptions in similar cases; first, because these remedies are not poisonous; second, because these reports are precisely the same kind of authority that physicians follow in making their prescriptions, and the same authority likewise that is relied upon by physicians in writing medical books, and that constitutes the foundation and largely the substance of the lectures to the students in medical colleges.

The names of diseases are retained here both because

they are in the articles cited and to aid the reader in iden-
tifying the *conditions* treated under those names.   The articles are considerably condensed for this place.

ABSCESS OF EAR.—Carrie A., age 16.   Severe pain in
left middle ear, with all the symptoms of gathering.   Calc.
Sulph., 3x, twice a day, cured in two days.—*The Homeo-*
pathic News.

ACCIDENT.—Clara M., 7 years.   Thrown and dragged
by a horse.   Left arm broken above elbow in two places,
about three inches apart ; left hand badly bruised ; right
arm and body bruised ; hoof-marks on face, right side of
which was crushed down ; head and neck swollen out an
inch ; both eyes closed ; mouth and tongue badly swollen.
I reached her one and a half hours after accident, and
found her in death-like stupor.   Gave Kali Phos., 3x,
every ten minutes, which banished the stupor.   Then gave
Kali Mur. and Ferrum Phos. alternately every fifteen minutes.   Set the arm under chloroform.   Second day gave
remedies every thirty minutes, and fourth day every hour.
Steady improvement from the first, and in three weeks
bandages were removed and she was dismissed a well girl.
Her life was saved by Ferrum Phos. and Kali Mur. in
large doses.—*J. C. Ferrell, M. D.*

ACUTE AILMENTS.—In mostly all acute ailments Ferr.
Phos. is absolutely the remedy to begin with, and if rightly
and early enough given will cut short the disease.   When
once exudation or suppuration has taken place, it is no
longer the indicated remedy, and we must look farther.
Still I would strongly advise the practitioner not to change
too quick from Ferrum Phos. to another remedy.   Be
cautious in this regard.—*Wm. Steinrauf, M. D.*

AFTER BIRTH, REMOVING.—Young lady, age 27.   The
labor was normal, but as soon as the child was expelled,

the uterus contracted with walls of abdomen hard, rigid and conical. I used several remedies to relax, but in vain. At last I gave Mag. Phos., fifteen grains (three doses in one), in hot water. In five minutes the relaxation occurred, and the placenta came away without further difficulty.— *Wm. Chapman, M. D.*

ANAEMIA.—Young lady, age 17. Became greatly debilitated ; had no appetite and no ambition ; her menses were irregular ; absent for months, then a flow varying in quantity. I gave her Calc. Phos., 6x, as principal remedy, also at times Ferrum Phos. as well. A few months and she was able to resume her studies.—*Dr. C. T. M.*

ANAEMIA.—Lizzie F,, age 16. Almost bloodless, nervous, almost strengthless, been so for months. Cured in five weeks with Calc. Phos., Kali. Phos. and a few doses of Kali. Mur.—*Dr. J. C. Ferrell.*

ASTHMA, CHRONIC.—Female, married, age 42. Subject to attacks for years ; expectoration greenish and remarkably copious. Natr. Sulph. every three hours. Improvement began after a few doses, expectoration becoming paler and less abundant ; has felt better since than for years ; and one noteworthy fact is, that the expectoration stopped in a few doses, whereas in previous attacks it had continued for weeks, thus indicating that the Natr. Sulph. had gotten at the root of the evil.—*Dr. Wm. J. Guernsey.*

ASTHMA, HUMID.—Old, chronic cases. In one instance respiration sounded like thin boiling mush. Two grains of Kali. Sulph , 3x, every two and a half hours has given me the most surprising results. I could ask for nothing better.—*Dr. G. W. Harvey.*

ASTHMA.—Young gentleman, J. G. Had been subject to severe attacks of asthma for several years. He tried Kali Phos. and Kali Mur., and experienced relief more quickly than by any other remedy he had tried.—*From Schuessler*.

BED-RIDDEN.—Miss R., age 24.   Left bed-ridden nine years ago from typhoid fever.   Has been treated by noted physicians of all schools.   I prescribed Kali Mur., 3x, two grains every six hours.   Improved at once, and in less than one year gained thirty-five pounds in weight, and is walking about without the assistance of a cane.— *V. W. Connor, M. D.*

BILIOUSNESS.—A case of bilious vomiting followed by voracious appetite, bitter taste and yellow skin.   I prescribed Nat. Sulph. for the biliousness, and Kali. Phos. for the appetite.   The second dose of Kali. Phos. relieved the stomach, and in forty-eight hours the skin was clear. This was after the quinine and pills of another physician had failed.—*F. S. Dunham, M. D.*

Another Case.—J. W., age 56.   Cutting pains in abdomen, bilious stools, coated tongue, yellow eyes and skin, heat in bowels, worse in damp weather.   Dr. H. S. Phillips prescribed Nat. Sulph., which resulted in speedy cure.

BITES FROM CENTIPEDE AND SCORPION.—Less than three grains of Nat. Mur. rubbed in with saliva on my little finger relieved me thoroughly in twenty minutes from the effects of the bite of a large centipede (five to six inches).

In scorpion bites, I suggest Ferrum Phos. in addition to Nat. Mur., should Nat. Mur. alone prove insufficient.— *Dr. C. V. Lorander.*

BLIND SPELLS AND HEADACHE.—Mr. B., engineer, age 59.   Blind spells, then flashy lights shooting out in rays and circles from one-half an hour to two hours, then an intense headache.   Come from once a day to once in three days.   Back head stiff and sore.   Troubled five years.   I gave Silica, 12x, and Calc. Flour, 3x, on alternate days, with occasionally Nat. Mur., 3x, and he was cured in three months.—*F. D. Bittinger, M. D.*

BRONCHITIS.—Lady Louisa has been subject to attacks of bronchitis for several winters, the first attack proving very serious. Ferrum Phos., a dose every hour, and a few doses of Kali. Phos. for exhausted condition, were steadily taken for a few days, and then Ferrum Phos. and Kali. Mur. alternately. The doctor who called to see her shortly after stated that the bronchial symptoms were all gone.—*Dr.* ———.

BRONCHITIS, CHRONIC.—Archibald Herbert, suffering from chronic bronchitis, had an attack of pneumonia ; had been exposed to great heat and took a chill and inflammation of right lung set in ; high fever, distressing cough, deep-seated pain in right side, expectoration tenacious, rusty colored. Ferrum Phos. in alternation with Kali. Mur., a dose every half hour, was taken for twenty-four hours ; then every hour. As the color of the sputa changed to yellow, he took Kali. Sulph. instead of Kali. Mur., and as this condition was remedied Nat. Mur. and Calc. Phos. completed the cure in a little more than ten days.—*Dr.* ———.

CANCER OF THE STOMACH.—Mrs. L., age 63, an Hebrew lady, came under my care suffering with sharp, lancinating pains in the stomach. External examination, cachexia, and all significant symptoms seemed to point to the one condition of cancer. In order to be sure of the diagnosis I took the liberty and precaution to have an examination made by two other physicians in whom I have great confidence, both of whom pronounced it cancer of the stomach, with the prognosis of course of the speedy termination of my patient's life. I remarked that I expected to get her up. My constant use of the Tissue Remedies has shown me what I can usually expect of them, and the remedies used were Cálc. Phos., 3x, in alternation with Kali. Phos., 3x ; a good-sized powder every three hours, until the cachexia and appearance of the face had changed to a more natural color, then I put her on Kali. Sulph., 6x. Nat. Mur., 6x, and Silica, 12x. In this order occasionally changing back to the Calc. Phos., Calc. Sulph., or Kali. Phos., as required by any change in her condition, and once or twice Nat. Phos. was used to quiet the pain.   In sixty days our patient was out of bed, and inside of ninety days she was out on the street, feeling as well as ever in her life.   She is alive and well to-day, and there has been no return of any symptoms that would lead us to suppose the whole trouble was not cured.—*F. D. Bittinger, M. D.*

CANCEROUS ULCER-EPITHELIOMA.—Wm. W., factory laborer.   Ulcer on right side of nose as large as a twenty-five cent piece ; been there four years ; eye much affected ; had been treated by two eye specialists and many physicians.   Dr. S. then took the case and gave Kali. Sulph. twice a day and a lotion of the same.   The inflammation disappeared in a few days'and the ulcer healed in a short time.

Another Case.—Miss A. D., age 20, had a similar sore on the left side of the nose, and of the same size, but had existed but six months and its center was covered with a horny scab, while the surrounding parts were just ready to ulcerate.   Dr. H. S. Phillips prescribed Kali. Sulph., 3x, every four hours, and a lotion of the same applied frequently.   The ulcer was cured in three weeks.

CARBUNCLE.—I have tried all (the recommended remedies) and must say that I am disgusted with them all. Now when I have a case of carbuncle I need nothing more than Silica. Give this internally and apply it locally, and your carbuncle will absolutely disappear without that destructive process which attends your incision or poultice methods.—*Dr. L. D. Foreman.*

CATARRH OF THE STOMACH.—My son, age 20, was confined to his bed four days with catarrh of the stomach ; had no appetite ; was very nervous with much pain in the stomach ; tongue coated with yellow, slimy deposit. I gave him Kali. Sulph., and after two doses there was a marked improvement, pain subsided and appetite returned.—*Dr. C. R. Taylor.*

CHILLS AND FEVER.—Nat. Mur. endears itself to the heart of the physician where this is such a common ailment, as it is more potent in those cases than any other one remedy.—*Dr. Frances McMillan.* (See Intermittent Fever).

CHILDREN, IMPERFECTLY FORMED.—The first child had a spine bifidia (cleft spine), club feet, womb prolapsed and protruding an inch externally. Lived two weeks. The mother never had been free from backache since she could remember. During her next pregnancy she took Calc. Phos., 5x, for seven months, and Sulphur. A perfect child without any trouble, even in dentition (teething), was the result, and two more children have been born under the same treatment whose only sickness has been mild scarlet fever, and the mother has no more backache.—*A. P. Macomber, M. D*

CHILDREN, UNDEVELOPMENT IN.—A tall, angular school marm, married at forty-two, brought to me the most scraggly, skinny and starved baby that I ever saw, of the neuter gender, several months old—her child, and bottle fed. I gave Calc. Phos., 6x. Three years later she called again and exclaimed, "Don't you know me? You saved my

boy's life.'' He improved from the very day that he began
the use of the medicine, and was then a fine healthy boy.
—*J. B. Chapman, M. D.*

CHILD BIRTH.—Fourth confinement, youngest child
eight years old, hard labor was expected. Gave Kali.
Phos., 3x, night and morning for six weeks, and it was the
easiest labor that I ever saw.—*D. Russell, M. D.*

CHILD BIRTH.—I was called to see a lady a week before confinement. Uneasy, restless, sleepless, with cutting,
flying pains some part of each day. I gave her Kali.
Phos. three times daily. No pain after taking the third
dose. Labor was almost painless. Gave birth to a fourteen pound girl. After the placenta was removed the
uterus did not contract readily and hemorrhage set in. I
gave Ferr. Phos. and Kali. Phos., 3x, alternately every
half hour, and in two hours the hemorrhage had ceased
and she recovered rapidly.—*Dr. M. McInnes.*

Second Case.—A very young person, sixteen years and
two months; very nervous and excited; did not know
what to expect; very much frightened. Gave her Kali.
Phos., 3x, every fifteen minutes; in an hour she was qui-
eted so as to sleep about three minutes between the contractions (pains) and everything was just perfect through-
out her lying-in.—*Dr. M. McInnes.*

CHOLERA INFANTUM.—Mary B., eighteen months old.
Green, watery stools, mixed with mucous, every few minutes, producing great weakness and emaciation. She
rolled her head about as if it was too heavy; eyes half
open; constant moaning or starting up in sleep; pulse
rapid; complexion of a dirty white appearance; watery
vomit. Ferrum Phos., 3x, in hot water, every hour for
six or eight times, then Calc. Phos. in alternation every

hour cured the case completely in less than one week.— *Dr.* ———.

COLIC, RENAL.—Was called to a case a few days ago who was suffering with most excruciating pain in the course of left ureter, vomiting, cold perspiration, cold extremities, small pulse, great agony, spasmodic cramping which would draw patient almost double, almost picture of death. Gave Mag. Phos., 3x, five grains in hot water, fifteen minutes repeated dose, the third relieved—patient was able to be up in less than two hours after first dose; next day was able to be at place of business. Who can say Mag. Phos. did not relieve?—*D. Russell, M. D.*

CONSTIPATION.—My twin brother wrote me in regard to his son, six years old. For the last year it has been almost impossible for him to have an action. Fecal matter would become impacted until it could not be passed without great pain. Had been so for over a year and under the doctor's care for months, but no better. I put the child on Silica, and after taking it five weeks he has had no further trouble. —*Dr. L. D. Foreman.*

COUGH, SPASMODIC.—Two cases. Worse at night und on lying down or breathing cold air; better sitting up; tightness of chest. One had spurting of urine when coughing. Both promptly relieved by Mag. Phos.—*Dr. F. W. Southworth.*

COUGH.—Mrs. B. caught cold, and it had settled on the lungs. Cough constantly, short, dry, inflammatory, hacking, and with considerable pain in the lungs. Gave Nat. Mur., 6x, and in less than an hour the cough had disappeared entirely and did not return. Ferr. Phos., 6x, and Nat. Mur., and in two days soreness in chest gone.—*Dr. J. B. Chapman.*

COUGH WITH EMISSIONS OF URINE.—A lady who was

suffering from a cough which caused great inconvenience, as with every cough there was emission of urine. Ferrum Phos. cured her speedily. A short time ago the lady, under similar circumstances, was again troubled with a cough. Ferrum. Phos. this time also cured her speedily.—*Dr. Fisher.*

CRAMP COLIC.—A stout man, age 45, florid, a high liver, doubled up with terrific cramps from eating heartily of boiled cabbage and ice cream on a hot day. Had such attacks frequently, and the wife said, "Nothing but morphine ever does John any good. Colocynth and other remedies failed. Then I gave Mag. Phos., 6x, in hot water every twenty minutes. The first dose relieved, and after the third he fell asleep.—*Dr. Frances McMillan.*

CRAMPS.—Mrs. M. R. S., age 61, severe cramps in bowels. Mag. Phos., four grains in hot water every half hour, relieved after two doses.—*M. F. Richards, M. D.*

CRAMPING AND DRAWING PAINS.—An experiment tried by Dr. G. L. Freemeyer was in his own case. He could find no remedies to relieve his cramping pains. Took seven doses of Mag. Phos., 2x, and has "not had a pain since." Result: "I now have a full set of the tissue (Biochemic) remedies, and prescribe them every day with good results."

CRAMPS, MENSTRUAL.—Mrs E. L. B. suffered with severe crampy pains at her periods. I used the biochemic remedies freely along with other treatment, and particularly Mag. Phos., 3x, a little before and during her period. She passed through without a particle of pain, and was so surprised and gratified she could not find words enough to express her thanks for the treatment received —*Dr. M. F. R.*

CROUP.—If taken in time, Ferrum Phos. and Kali. Mur.

is all that is required.. A gargle of Kali. Mur. is very beneficial, when practicable.—*Dr.* ———.

CROUP, MEMBRANOUS.—Severe case. Treatment was Ferrum Phos., 3x, twenty grains dissolved in one-half glass of water, a teaspoonful every half hour or an hour, as case demanded. I did not try to reduce the fever at once—as I think fever is one of our best friends in disease. The little patient had a very dry, distressed breathing, what might be called a "spongia cough." For this I knew that the fibrin must not be allowed to remain in the diseased parts ; consequently I used twenty grains of Kali. Mur. to one-half glass of water, and ordered teaspoonful given every seven, fifteen or twenty minutes as was needed to keep him in a nice breathing condition. I used a table napkin squeezed out of cold water and changed on his neck as soon as it got warm. This cured the worst case of membranous croup I have seen in twenty years.—*Dr. G. F. Dougherty.*

- CROUP, MEMBRANOUS,—One of my children is subject to membranous croup, and Kali. Mur., 3x, always controls it better than anything I have ever given.—*Dr. L. D. Foreman.*

CROUPY COUGH.—Five powders of Kali. Mur., 2x, cured a case that had been under allopathic and eclectic treatment (five) days.—*G. L. Freemeyer, M. D.*

CROUP, SPURIOUS.—D. R., a boy of seven years, who took spurious croup whenever there was a sharp, keen, northeast wind, having had, a few years before, a very severe attack of true croup, this autumn had again an attack with fever and a loud, barking cough. I gave every two hours a full dose of Kali. Mur. After a few doses the cough became loose, lost completely the barking sound,

and the following morning my patient was able to get up.
—*D. Schuessler.*

CYSTITIS (inflammation of bladder).—This is a very frequent trouble, and one that has given me no small amount
of anxiety, until I began the use of the Tissue Remedies.
In the treatment of cystitis I find in asthenic conditions
with prostration, frequent urination with excessive secretion of urine or passing of blood in the urine, Kali. Phos.
is the remedy in the 6x; it will not disappoint you in a
single case.   When we have retention and frequent desire
to urinate with spasmodic conditions, drawing and pull-
ing sensation, I would advise you to give Mag. Phos.
with confidence.   I have been using the Schuessler Tissue remedies for a number of years in these affections and I
find them first-class in every respect.—*G. F. Dougherty,
M. D.*

DECLINE.—Gertie I, age 18.   "Languid, listless, stupid, tired all over, poor appetite and menses every two
weeks," was her mother's description.   Fever, dry, coated
tongue, backache and suspected typhoid also.   Gave Baptisia three days, no better.   Gave Gels. with same result.
Then gave Calc. Fluor., and the change was to me mar-
velous in its suddenness and completeness.—*H. S. Phillips, M. D.*

DELIRIUM TREMENS.—Speedily cured by Nat. Mur.—
Walker.

DIARRHEA, ARMY.—An old soldier afflicted with spells
of it ever since the war.   Was reduced to skin and bones
almost, no appetite, seemed like the last call.   A few days
treatment with Nat. Mur., 6x, made him feel as if he had
been resurrected.— *D. L. Hurd, M. D.*

DIARRHEA, INFANTILE.—Child, 3 weeks old, screaming
with pain; green, slimy discharge.   The pains were soon

relieved with Mag. Phos. and the discharges arrested by Nat. Sulph.—*D. L. Hurd, M. D.*

DIARRHEA AND FEVER.—Child, 18 months old, temperature 104°, pulse 130°, face flushed, nerves excited, eyes staring, great thirst, frequent green, slimy evacuations, vomiting, pain in stomach and abdomen. Ordered one grain of Ferr. Phos. and Mag. Phos. every thirty minutes in alternation. Began to feel relief from the first dose, was sleeping nicely in two hours and rapidly recovered.—*W. E. Kinnett, M. D.*

DIPTHERIA.—Under the regular treatment was so severe that the physician in charge gave up all hope of recovery and another physician was called. He gave Ferrum Phos. and Kali. Mur. and the case recovered. This is only one case of several that I can mention where the Tissue Remedies have most nobly asserted themselves. I believe that Biochemistry is yet in its infancy, and when it is understood and used by all I cannot help thinking and saying, Oh! what will the harvest be?—*Dr. A. P. Betts.*

DIPTHERIA.—Miss H., age 16. High fever, rapid pulse and soreness in throat and upper part of chest; both tonsils covered with a white exudation about the size of the ball of the thumb; tongue white; restless, sleepless, etc. Prescribed Ferrum Phos. and Kali. Mur. in alternation every hour, and a gargle of Kali. Mur. to be used frequently. Improvement was immediate and a good recovery was made in four or five days.—*Dr. J. B. Chapman.*

DIPTHERIA.—October 16th Master S., a bright, scholarly boy of 14, pain in back of head, temperature 102½. I deferred diagnosis, but gave Ferrum Phos. for the fever.

Oct. 17th. Symptoms all worse; gray spots on both tonsils, and diptheritic odor. Diagnosis: diptheria. Prescribed ten grains each Ferr. Phos. and Kali. Mur., 3x, in two glasses half full of water; a teaspoonful every half hour, alternately.

Oct. 18th. Great extension of membrane to both tonsils and uvula. 'Remedies as before, and in addition twenty grains Kali. Mur. in a tumbler of water for gargling every three or four hours.

Oct. 19th. Tonsils and uvula thickly covered with dark, cadaverous-smelling membrane, which had also invaded, posterior nares. Gave Ferrum Phos., Kali. Mur. and Kali. Phos., alternately, every half hour.

Oct. 20th. Hoarse, croupal cough and great difficulty in respiration, showing that membrane had descended into the larynx. Membrane protruding from both nostrils, which exuded a thin excoriating ichor. Total inability to breathe through nose. Patient had several attacks of epistaxis (nose bleed) during night. Unendurable stench from mouth. For the nose bleed I put thirty drops of Crotalus Hor., 10x, in water, and gave a teaspoonful three or four times. Remedies: Kali. 'Mur., Kali. Phos. and Calc. Phos.

Oct. 21st. Several attacks of nose bleed; no improvement except that there was little fever. Remedies as before. Added to the gargle one-third alcohol. The boy used this freely, as he found it helped breathing.

Oct. 22d. Membrane beginning to soften and peel off from the anterior portion of the tonsils. But little epistaxis to-day. Continued remedies.

Oct. 23d. Marked improvement; patient spit out large sloughs of membrane. Continued remedies.

Oct. 24th. Great improvement; no more nose bleed; boy able to breathe a little through left nostril; though he spit out a great deal of dark membrane, there is still plenty in trachea. Remedies as before.

Oct. 25th. Tonsils, uvula and larynx, as far as visible, clean; no bleeding of surfaces; both nostrils free; still hoarse and talked with difficulty, but respiration easy. Remedies: Kali. Phos. and Calc. Phos.

Oct. 26th. Patient practically dismissed; when he got up he had paralysis of vocal chords and very great asthenopia, but Kali Phos., 2 gr. four times a day for a couple of weeks restored them to the normal condition.

On the fifth day of this boy's sickness his sister, six years old, was taken with the same disease. Ferr. Phos. and Kali Mur. were all the remedies she took, as her attack was not so violent. I had eight other cases in the immediate neighborhood: none were virulent; all treated and cured with Kali. Mur. and Ferr. Phos. There were quite a number of deaths under "regular" treatment.— *Dr. A. C. Davis.*

DIPTHERIA.—In fourteen cases of diptheria the biochemic measures left nothing better to be desired, Kali. Mur. rapidly making a change; the whitish-gray exudations being diminished, shriveling and coming away with the gargle and mouth-wash made with Kali. Mur., also occasional doses of Ferr. Phos. The treatment worked splendidly. In three cases the patients labored under prostration from the first, and Kali. Phos. had to be given inter currently; in two cases Nat. Mur. alternately with Kali. Mur., the chief remedy. In the latter cases there existed considerable running of saliva, heavy drowsiness and watery stools No secondary affection resulted, such as frequently arise under ordinary treatment; as paralysis, defective vision or neuralgia.—*Dr. Walker.*

DIPTHERIA.—Son of H. T. L. Malignant diptheria,

temperature 104, pulse 140. Ferr. Phos., 3x, every hour, and Kali. Mur., 6x, every hour. Two days later kidneys involved. Calc. Phos., 3x, in rotation with the other. Temperature 99, pulse 100, throat nearly clean. Dropped Ferr. Phos. and Calc. Phos. and gave Kali. Mur., 3x, and Nat. Mur., 6x, and the next day discharged the case cured. —*S. M. Kessler, M. D.*

DISPLACEMENTS, UTERINE.—I have made a specialty of this disease (displacement) for a number of years, and my experience is, that the judicious use of Biochemic remedies, combined with the nightly replacing of the uterus, will give better satisfaction than any other system known. —*Dr. J. B. Chapman.*

[His method of replacing is very simple, is accomplished by the patient unaided, and with a slight improvement is as follows, viz.. After retiring, take the knee-chest position, i. e., resting on knees with chest on the flat bed, not on pillow, with both hands draw the bowels forward, then insert one forefinger into the vagina and press up against the perineum (the tissue between the vagina and anus) thus filling the vagina with air, which will operate as a cushion or tampon. Then gently lie down on the back if the displacement is forward, on the chest if it is backward, and with the foot of the bed elevated on blocks eight inches if it is downward. Turn to any natural position when tired. Do this every night, and if practicable at a forenoon and afternoon rest also ; certainly at one rest time in the day. To strengthen the ligaments, take Calc. Fluor four times a day, and during two to six of the most active hours of the day wear a pledget of cotton saturated with Calc. Fluor—ten doses to the ounce of soft water—pressed up against the uterus and held in place by dry sterilized wool packed in the vagina, but not uncomfortably full.

Calc. Phos. and Kali. Phos., one dose of each one to three times a day in uncomplicated cases, as constitutional and nerve tonics. Other salts if indicated by complications. Keep bowels soft with colon flush of hot water three to seven times a week].

DYSMENORRHEA (painful menstruation).—Young lady, age 20, had been' troubled every month since puberty with almost unbearable pains in uterus, back and loins, beginning several hours before the flow and continuing two days. The second day hysterical fits came on, and on the third relief from pain. I found her almost mad with pain. Gave Mag. Phos. every ten minutes, and in an hour the pain ceased. Ordered two doses a day for three days. The next month ordered three doses the day before the period and every three hours the first day. Had but slight pain. Repeated the same prescription the third month; no pain, and none since.—*Homeopathic World*.

DYSMENORRHEA.—Patient in bed, pains seemed unbearable. Had been troubled so every month. I gave Mag. Phos., repeated in half an hour. In a short time she was easy.—*D. Russell, M. D.*

DYSPEPSIA, FERMENTIVE.—Nat. Phos., 3x or 6x, in fermentive dyspepsia will control it better than any one drug. —*Dr. L. D. Foreman.*

EAR PAIN.—Mrs. B. had much swelling and redness and *very* severe pain of middle left ear. Gave Mag. Phos. and Ferr. Phos. that night with no good result. Next morning changed to Calc. Sulph., 3x, and the second dose gave relief, and in twenty-four hours the redness and swelling were gone.—*Dr. D. Russell.*

EAR TROUBLES.—I think it is the best remedy in the Materia Medica in diseases of the ear—Kali. Mur. In chronic catarrhal conditions of the middle ear, noises in the ear, snapping sensation, deafness or earache from swelling of the eustachian tube, and cracking noise on swallowing or blowing the nose, with aurists of all schools it is a standard medicine.—*Dr. Wm. Steinrauf.*

EPILEPTIC CONVULSIONS.—A girl about 16 years of age. Convulsions began when menses first appeared, and harder and more frequently in spite of all remedies, until she had them several times a day. My wife prescribed Calc. Phos. and Kali. Phos. in alternation. She took them, and never had but one convulsion after that, fully regained her health and is now stout and strong.—*Dr. C. W. Cramer.*

ERYSIPELAS OF FACE.—I have treated three very pronounced cases of erysipelas of the face and head with Ferr. Phos., one grain every hour, and a cloth wet in a solution of the same constantly applied. Also used internally Nat. Sulph. I was surprised at the ameliorations of the disease. The cures were more rapid than by any other treatment that I have ever used.— *W. E. Kinnett, M. D.*

ERYSIPELAS OF ARM AND FACE.—H. B., age 60, bruised left arm near elbow. Five days later pain and burning set in. On the seventh day when I was called, found arm extremely inflamed and swollen, and by scratching it and his nose it had been transferred to the face. Nat. Sulph. and Kali. Mur. alternately every two hours. Fourth day itching and pain gone, redness nearly gone, place scaly. Changed to Kali. Sulph. every three hours, and on the sixth day of treatment was well.—*H. G. Merz, M. D.*

EYES, INFLAMMATION OF.—Little Etta B., age 2. The ball almost a scarlet red, considerable pain and great intolerance of light. Ferr. Phos. quickly relieved, and the third stage, with discharge of thick yellow matter, Calc. Sulph., alternated with Ferr. Phos., satisfactorily removed. —*Dr. J. B. C.*

FELONS.—A dressmaker had a felon on right thumb. Ferr. Phos., 12x, every three hours promptly cured it as she thought, but much use caused its reappearance in three days with greatly increased pain and swelling. Kali. Mur. finished the cure at once.—*Dr. J. C. Morgan.*

FEET SWEATING.—A. J., age 16, had been troubled with foot-sweat for two months; could wear his stockings only one day, and at night would be wringing wet; the odor was something awful; his shoes became so saturated with sweat, and the odor was so foul, that, when he took them off at night, one could scent them in any part of the room, and even in adjoining rooms; his feet became sore and tender. I gave Sil., 3x, a powder three times a day. In a week his feet began to show signs of improvement, and in a short time were completely cured.—*Chironian.*

FEVER, INTERMITTENT.—Mr. H., age 27, had chills every third day from 9 to 11 A. M., with violent headache, great thirst, followed by fever from about 1 P. M. to evening, accompanied by great lassitude, increased headache and thirst, profuse, sour-smelling sweat, and loss of appetite. Twelve powders of Nat. Mur., 6x, failed to relieve. Then gave three powders of Nat. Mur., 200x, one every other night. Cured in two weeks, and no return of disease in eight months.—*Dr. C. R. Vogel.*

Another Case.—Mrs. M., age 32. Sanguine temperament, nervous and irritable. Chilly all the time, but worse about 3 A. M.; great hunger; fever at its height about 2 P. M.; intense thirst; short, difficult breathing and profuse perspiration Silica, 6x, a powder night and morning for one week cured.—*Dr. C. R. Vogel.*

FEVER, INTERMITTENT.—Nat. Mur. will cure more cases of intermittent fever, both acute and chronic, especially the latter, than any other remedy in the Materia Medica —*Dr. Burt.*

FEVER, TYPHO-MALARIAL.—Wm. H., age 25. Temperature 103.4°, pulse 99. Gave Ferr.' Phos. and Kali. Phos. alternately every hour. Third day temperature 103°, pulse 80. Gave the remedies every two hours. Fourth day temperature 101°, pulse 80. Three days later temperature suddenly rose to 103°. Gave the remedies again every hour for three days, when it was under control. Four days later he came to my office as well as ever in his life.—*H. G. Merz, M. D.*

FEVER, TYPHO-MALARIAL.—Johnnie L., age 8, treated the first week with Baptisia ; second week, Ferr. Phos. alternated with Kali. Phos. ; fever gone on the twelfth day. Relapse three days later, cured in five weeks by Ferr. Phos. and Kali. Phos., with an occasional dose of Calc. Phos., with no hemorrhage, and very rapid convalescence. —*John M. Reid, M. D.*

FEVER, TYPHOID.—Mrs. B., age 25. Had been sick two weeks, and given up to die by two prominent allopathic physicians. Had been kept on boiled milk for ten days. She begged for grapes and pears. I gave them as almost her sole diet for the next week. For her watery discharges every few minutes I gave Nat. Sulph. Kali. Phos. for weakness, emaciation and typhoid condition. Ferr. Phos. for fever, from one-half to one hour apart. When stools changed, gave Kali. Mur. Improvement began at once, and she made a perfect recovery.— *Wm. Chapman, M. D.*

GALL-STONE COLIC.—Mrs. T., age 36. A paroxysm every other night for six months ; getting worse ; one to two hours of agony each time ; breathing hard and tight : face red and swollen ; extremities clammy ; pulse slow.

Allopathic physicians gave morphine hypodermic injections and wanted to operate surgically. I gave Mag. Phos., 2x, dissolved in hot water as a hypodermic injection three times, and Nat. Mur., 6x, in teaspoonful doses every five minutes for an hour, then every half hour until she slept. The next day Kali. Mur., 6x, and next Nat. Mur. This day she had a light attack, which was stopped by one hypodermic of Mag. Phos. Three days later was threatened with another, which was warded off by simply keeping feet in hot water. No return of the disease; but continued the medicine about two months.—*F. D. Bittenger, M. D.*

GUM BOIL.—Lily, 6 years old, had an ulcerated tooth with a well-developed gum boil. Gum boil would not go away, and wishing to see what the Tissue Salts would do for it, I gave her a Christmas present of a box containing about 125 tablets of Calcarea Sulph., 3x. They should have lasted her ten days or more, but they were sweet, and so the box was gone in three days. And so was the gum boil and ulcerated tooth. Neither have troubled her since. In this you will perceive a first-class recommendation for the Biochemic Tablets. They are pleasant to take. An old German lady once said to me respecting them, "These are the bestest pills I ever took."—*Dr. M. F. Richards.*

HEADACHE.—A lady subject to this affliction. Frequent; worse in damp weather; apt to occur the day after her weekly washing of clothes; comes on gradually in morning and lasts all day. Symptoms: Hard, pressive aching with occasional heat in vertex; markedly better on lying down; vertigo on suddenly turning the head. I administered one dose, a five-grain powder of Calc. Phos., 6x, dry on the tongue, and the headache entirely disappeared in half an hour.—*Dr. A. E. Barrett.*

HEADACHE.—A rush of blood to the head, with a fiery red face, often vomiting, and is worse on stooping. Ferr. Phos. cured — *Wm. Steinrauf, A. M., M. D.*

HEART PAINS.—Miss M. was seized with excessive pains of the heart, so severe that she lost consciousness. Under treatment the pains were somewhat mitigated, but remained severe at times for twenty-four hours. Magnes. Phos. gave entire relief with a few doses. A little soreness remained, but Ferrum Phos. cleared it up in a few hours. —*Dr. ———.*

HEART PANGS —I was called one night to see Capt. G——, age 56, who was suffering severely with heart trouble. I found him with very weak pulse—forty-two beats to the minute—sharp, darting, intense pains in the heart, so that he breathed with great difficulty. I mixed him Kali. Phos., 6x, in hot water. Immediately thereafter he began gulping spasmodically. Magnes. Phos., 6x, stopped it at once—he not making one single gulp after taking the remedy. Under Magnes. Phos. and Kali. Phos. in alternation the pulse rose from forty-two to sixty-four in ten minutes. The pains ceased, and he made a most rapid recovery. Magnes. Phos. has frequently proven itself one of the best anti-pain and anti-spasmodic remedies known to the medical world. It not only does the required work promptly and effectually, but is entirely harmless, leaving no train of after effects.— *Wm. Chapman, M. D.*

HEMORRHAGE FROM LUNGS.—The blood was bright red and coagulated almost as soon as discharged. Gave Ferr. Phos., 2x, five grains every half hour. Results good.— *The Homœopathic News.*

HYDROCEPHALUS, TO PREVENT.—A mother whose husband had old-fashioned, many years lasting consumption, had lost four children with hydrocephalus. I recommended Calc. Phos., 5x, during the next pregnancy. She took it from the seventh week until her confinement. The bones of the child's head were more perfect than those of his body. In eighteen months, another fine healthy boy was added to the family, she having taken the same treatment during pregnancy. After my first call to the dying fourth child, I was the physician of the family for ten years, but was never called for the two boys but once. The father died two years after the birth of the second.—*A. P. Macomber, M. D.*

INCONTINENCE OF URINE —Three cases have been completely relieved by the use of Silica —*Dr.* ———.

INSANITY, OCCASIONAL —Miss M., daughter of Dr. M., had suffered for several years from occasional attacks of insanity, which grew worse until it was thought necessary to send her to an asylum. A friend interposed and urged the trial of the Biochemic remedies. Kali. Phos., four doses a day, were given for weeks, and completely cured her. Several cases of a similar nature, two of them puerperal mania, have been treated with equal success.— *Schuessler.*

INFLUENZA,—Mr. R., age 26. Bookkeeper; perfectly well in morning; about 10 o'clock very tired and weak; considerable sneezing and much lachrymation, with thin, watery discharge from nares. Temperature the following two days was 103 to 104. Great soreness of muscles, severe backache and bone pains, and pain in throat up to ear when swallowing. I prescribed the usual homeopathic remedies, Gelsem. and Euper. Per., but did not get any perceptible results. Discharge now a profuse, greenish mucous, with much accumulated in throat and mouth. I then prescribed Nat. Sulph., 6x, every hour, about five grains at a dose. The result was striking. In a few hours he felt so much better that it was with difficulty he was kept in the house. The following morning he went to work, and has not been troubled any more with influenza. —*Dr. H. LaDerne.*

INDIGESTION.—Child 10 years old under doctor's care two weeks without benefit. Had indigestion from over-study and worry, with brown tongue. Kali. Phos., 3x, every hour started her on the road to recovery at once. Appetite returned in twenty-four hours. Well in four days.—*Dr. M. F. R.*

INFLAMMATION OF THE MASTOID CELLS —Mr. F., age 30 years, had what he called neuralgia, located posterior to the left ear, pain constant of a cutting, darting nature. I called it inflammation of the mastoid cells, and gave him Ferrum Phos , 3x, and Silica, 4x, cautioning him to see me when the medicine was out. After a few days he said he was all right and needed no further treatment. Then in fifteen days he came back with a swelling as large as an orange, very painful and hard to the touch. I gave him Ferrum Phos. and Silica as before, and in a little over a month he was sound and well.—*Dr. E. Jas. Milvain.*

INTERMITTENT NEURALGIA.—Mrs. S., age 49. Inter-mittent neuralgia; lost rest several nights. I gave Mag-nes. Phos. in hot water every five minutes; pain gone in twenty minutes.—*Dr. M. H. White.*

LABOR.—"In labor, when the pains are too weak and irregular, I have seen nothing act more promptly and effectually than Kali. Phos."—*Dr. E. H. Holbrook.*

LAGRIPPE—INFLUENZA.—All cases treated by me with Nat. Sulph. were free from any evil after-effects whatever. The after-effects in cases treated by other physicians with other remedies were cured by this salt.—*Dr. Schuessler.*

LAGRIPPE.—Carrie M., age 16. Profuse discharges

from the nares (nostrils.) Pains of a rheumatic nature, involving the muscles of the limbs and joints; chilly, with high, continuous temperature; tongue coated white; great depression; felt as though she had been sick for months. Kali. Mur. 3x, every two hours, cured in three days.—*Dr. Chas. F. Wright.*

LaGrippe.—I have found that Nat. Sulph. will serve the greater number of cases, and have received wonderful results from its use. both at the beginning and when followed by sequelæ (effects of the disease).—*Chas. S. Vaught, M. D.*

Laryngitis and Tonsilitis, Acute.—Mr. P., age 50, an old soldier, voice husky and hoarse, cough irritating and painful, nearly croupy, dry, much pain in larynx and throat, and constriction of upper chest, tonsils dark red, much swollen, filled with ulcerations, pulse 100, temperature 102½. Gave Ferr. Phos. 15 grains in one-half glass of water, a teaspoonful every hour. In 24 hours the fever was gone, in two days tonsils clean and in four days from the first dose he resumed business.—*J. Ferris, M. D.*

He also details the case of Mrs. D., quite similar to the above, cured in three days by the same remedy.

Leucorrhea —Minne S., age 17, suffered with an acrid, albuminous, tenacious leucorrhea, worse after periods. Gave Calc. Phos., 3x, every four hours, and every other day a douche of non-alcoholic Calendula. Cured in a short time —*The Homeopathic News.*

On May 30th I was called upon to prescribe for a little girl four years of age. Since birth she had been troubled with a very offensive vaginal discharge. Many physicians had been employed, but had entirely failed to benefit the case. The discharge was very profuse—yellow, " like sulphur"—the mother explained—fœted odor—and caused rawness and soreness wherever it touched the flesh.

Her appetite was poor—bowels constipated, and there were symptoms of worms, although none had been seen. I prescribed Kali Sulph. and Nat. Phos., 15 grains, in a glass half full of water, taken by small sips during the day; the Kali. Sulph. one day and the Nat. Phos. the next, and so on.   After one month's treatment the child was no better, and I began to think that I should go the way of my predecessors.

I now made a more thorough examination, and discovered there was a syphilitic history on the mother's side. On examination the teeth plainly showed the disease.

I now changed the treatment to Kali. Mur. 3x, and as there were still worm symptoms the Nat. Phos. 3x was continued.   I also gave intercurrent doses of Calc. Phos. 6x on general principles.   I gave medicine enough for two weeks, and as *two months* went by and I heard nothing more of the case, I supposed that another physician was trying his hand at it.   What was my surprise last night when the mother came to pay her account and reported that the child was *entirely* well—" not a drop of discharge "—no worm symptoms—in fact every abnormal symptom gone and the child well and happy.

I am inclined to give the credit to the Kali. Mur., assisted by the Calc. Phos., but still, one cannot say positively that the other remedies did not assist—but this I do know for certain : that one or more of these four biochemic remedies were responsible for the cure, as nothing else was given.—*Dr. J. B. Chapman.*

MALARIA.—T. W., an old sailor, cutting pains in abdomen and left hypochrondriac region.   Bilious stools, worse in damp weather, heat in bowels and rectum, gastric derangement, coated tongue, yellow conjunctiva, sallow skin. Had suffered from malaria in former years, and now resides on the river bank, a low, damp, miasmatic region.

Had prescribed for him several times before receiving the tissue remedies without avail. I prescribed Natrum Sulph. The result was speedy and most satisfactory. That was four months ago, and he informed me yesterday that he has been free from pain ever since, and never felt better in his life.—*Dr. H. S. Phillips.*

MENORRHAGIA (Excessive menstrual flow).—Mrs. A., æt. thirty-four; profuse menstruation of bright red blood every three, sometimes every two weeks, lasting from five to six days. Small, thin, anæmic; face pale; during the menstrual period just the reverse—face livid, ofttimes of a fiery red, with much heat and burning. Blood coagulates as soon as expelled from uterus, clotting in the vagina. Vomits everything she eats; debility. Ferr. Phos. every two hours during the period, and night and morning for a week. This treatment was continued for about three months, when the flow became more normal, her complexion better, and she began to feel stronger and much improved in every way.—*Dr.*———.

MENSTRUATION DELAYED.—In young girls with flushed cheeks, headache and backache, so happy have been the results of use of Ferr. Phos. that it is almost the first remedy I think of in such cases.—*Dr. Frances McMillan.*

MENSTRUATION—PAINFUL.—For the cramping in painful menstruation Mag. Phos. has given me more satisfaction than all the Blue Cohosh and Pulsatilla I ever gave. —*Dr. L. D. Foreman.*

MENSTRUATION—PAINFUL.—Young lady, age 18, had painful periods for five years. Her screams could be heard

two blocks away for nearly two days.   Ferr. Phos. and
Kali Phos. were given in alternation.   The next period
was nearly free from pain, the second quite free, and all
other bad symptoms fast disappearing.—*J. B. Chapman,
M. D.*

I had a call from a lady who was the wife of an allo-
path.   Said she: " Doctor, I suppose you think it very
strange for me to call on you for treatment when you
know my husband is a physician, and practicing medicine also ; but, Doctor, I am troubled with painful and
scanty menstrual periods, and I almost die every month,
and I guess I would if it were not for the Morphine that
the doctor gives me to numb the pain.   I have met so
many of my lady acquaintances and heard them say that
you gave them relief so quickly, I resolved to pick up the
courage and call on you for some medicine for that particular difficulty ; but you will do me a great favor by
keeping this a secret, so that my husband won't get hold
of it."

And I promised to do so, and I shall, unless he by
chance should read this article, and if he should, I think
it might set him to thinking and he would drop the Morphine and try the tissue remedies instead of making light
of them.—*G. L. Freemyer, M. D.*

P. S.—Gave her Kali. Phos. and Ferr. Phos., which relieved her.   Has been all O. K. ever since.

NECROSIS (Rotting of bone):—A lady had some teeth
removed by a dentist, and instead of getting better, grew
worse, and there was a continual discharge from the
cavity.   The gum around the bone was purple and offensive.   I gave her Silica and Calc. Fluorica, 6x.   In less
than two months the discharge had entirely ceased, and
she was much better.—*Dr. Farrington.*

NERVOUSNESS AND IRREGULARITY.—Mrs. K., age 32, very nervous, emaciated, weak, poor appetite, constant worry, menses profuse every fourteen days, acrid secretions, and cold and numb extremities: Cured in four weeks by Kali. Phos. and Calc. Phos.—*Dr. H. P.*

NEURALGIA OF UTERUS AND OVARIES.—In such cases Mag. Phos. gives almost magical relief.—*Dr. Frances Mc-Millan.*

NEURALGIA.—Miss Margaret S., suffered from neuralgia, true nerve fibre pain darting through her head along the nerves. She had suffered intermittently for three days. Two doses of Mag. Phos. cured her completely.—*Dr.* ———

NEURALGIC HEADACHE.—Mrs. K——— had a slight hoarseness, but otherwise did not feel indisposed. She began her spring house cleaning rather early, worked in cold rooms, and what with the cold, dust, and hard work, was taken one afternoon with a high fever, accompanied with a severe headache. She took Ferrum Phos. and Kali. Mur. alternately in three grain doses every hour, and also several hot foot baths, and at night a cathartic pill. In the morning fever gone, but headache remained; when standing, head seemed too full, ached on top, and all around base; heat to the head seemed more relieving than cold. I took from twelve to eighteen tablets each of Kali. Phos., Nat. Phos. and Mag. Phos., dissolved them in two-thirds of a glass of water, and told her to take a teaspoonful every fifteen minutes until all was taken, or she felt relieved. In five hours headache was gone, and she was up and around the house. I should add that she took a hot foot bath and kept a hot water bag to her feet.—*Dr. M. F. Richards.*

NIGHT SWEATS.—Mr. P., a teamster, broad-chested,

strong and healthy, would wake in the night and find himself drenched with sweat.   I gave him Silica, 6x, five or six grains morning and evening.   A week later, and the sweats had left him and did not return.—*Dr.*———

NON-ASSIMILATION.—Old man about 60.   Dyspepsia, the doctors said.   Emaciated, pale, swarthy ; no appetite ; restless ; bowels inactive ; stools sometimes light-colored, and at times costive ; tongue thickly coated with a brownish yellow tinge ; bitter taste ; conjunctiva a blueish white ; skin wrinkled and bowels retracted and shrunken, shriveled, and a pain in the stomach of a burning character after eating ; and from the general character of the case, assimilation was greatly at fault.   The man had been, and was at that time, taking Argentum, in pill form, from a "regular," three doses a day, and had been for a year or more ; all to no purpose, except to hasten the emaciation. I at once put him on Nat. Sulph , 6x, three doses a day before meals, and Kali. Phos., 6x, as a nerve remedy.   These two remedies perfectly cured the "dyspepsia" and all the other troubles, so that in about three weeks he was a well man, the Nat. Sulph. correcting all the liver and stomach troubles, and the Kali. Phos. building up the nerve forces. —*Dr. A. P. Davis.*

ORCHITIS (inflammation of testicles).—Mr. J.   Caused by chafing from riding bicycle.   Right testicle about four times normal size ; pulse over 100 ; Movement caused pain. Ferrum Phos., 6x, and Kali. Mur., 3x, alternately every hour.   A cold sitz bath at 75 degrees, three times a day, for one minute, and return to bed without thoroughly drying.   In three days was able to be up by using a suspensory, and in one week all right.—*M. F. Richards, M. D.*

PAIN IN BACK, COUGH, ETC.—A lady had pain in her back clear across just below the shoulder blades for several months ; also nervous, pain in lower lobe of right lung, and worrying cough. I prescribed Ferr. Phos. and Kali. Mur. with Calc. Phos. intercurrently. This removed the cough and soreness of lung, but the pain in back was worse. Learning that she had had a severe mental strain, I then placed her upon Kali. Phos., 3x, twenty grains in a glass half full of water, a teaspoonful every hour (equivalent to five grains an hour. S. H. P.). This was repeated each day for a week, when her pain was entirely gone.—*Dr. J. B. C.*

PARALYSIS.—Mr. J. D., age 70. Lay as if dead, with whole right side paralyzed. Gave one grain of Kali. Phos. every hour. In a few weeks was up and around, and continues rapidly improving, seven weeks after attack.— *W. E. Kinnett, M. D.*

PARALYSIS, FACIAL.—Henry K., age 24. Right side of face paralyzed ; walked with shuffling gait ; hands and feet cold, and would occasionally shake as if with palsy. Kali. Phos., 3x, and Calc. Phos., 3x, in alternation every three hours for two weeks, then Kali. Phos. alone. In three months is nearly cured.—*Dr. C. R. Vogel.*

PARALYSIS OF THE VOCAL CHORDS.—A young lady about 18 years awoke one morning, found that she could whisper only, otherwise she didn't think there was anything wrong with her. She consulted her physician, but received no help. After this I saw her. She didn't whisper, but sometimes spoke hoarse. I gave Kali. Phos., 6x, about five grains in six spoonsful of water, to be taken every day. The second day improvement began, and soon had her voice again.—*Dr. Wm. Lenz.*

PEMPHIGUS (blisters on the skin).—A baby, age 10 months. Watery blisters covering all the genital region, and extending down the thighs and up as far as the navel, which were of various sizes, from that of a pea to a large walnut. Upon breaking them they discharged a thin, watery, colorless fluid, and after collapsing left a dry but inflamed scar. A considerable itching, but otherwise health as usual. I prescribed Nat. Mur , 6x, fifteen· grains dissolved in twelve teaspoonsful of water   Dose: One teaspoonful an hour apart, while awake. The blisters stopped coming, those present dried up and only scars remained.—*Dr. J. B. C.*

PERITONITIS AND OVARITIS, CHRONIC (inflammation of ovaries and lining membrane of the abdomen).—Mrs. E., age 38, had suffered thus many years. For a severe aggravation, Dr. G. H. Martin gave Ferr. Phos. every fifteen minutes for two hours, then every hour for several days. She then removed, but after two years has never had the slightest symptoms of her old trouble.

PILES.—Wm. S., age 28. Troubled for some years with bleeding piles, constipation, pressure of blood to head, flushes of heat, tongue mapped or covered with a grayish white coating. Calc. Fluor., 3x, and Kali. Mur., 6x, in alternation every four hours, with an ointment ·of Calc. Fluor., 2x, one-half ounce to vaseline two ounces, and applied locally every night completely cured him in a few weeks.— *The Homœopathic News.*

PNEUMONIA.—The worst case that I ever saw was relieved beautifully in a few hours after the best selected remedies had failed for days, by Ferr. Phos. There was complete consolidation of the left lung and of the lower lobe of the right with a strong tendency to complete of the right; temperature 103° to 104°; most rapid pulse, and an agony of pain and rapid respiration. The fever left and the pulse steadied in a few days. Suppuration ensued, for the Ferr. Phos. was not administered early

enough to prevent it, but he made a good recovery.—*Dr.*
———.

PNEUMONIA.—Robert R., a stout plethoric Scotchman,
age 30. Intense inflammation of lungs, high fever, tightness of chest, labored breathing, dry skin, racking cough
without expectoration, aching all over and a beating headache. Ordered hot sponge bath, hot injections, spice bag
to chest, and Ferr. Phos., 3x, and Kali. Mur., 3x, four
tablets (one grain) every hour alternately. The day after the cough was loose with abundant white expectoration streaked with blood, perspiring, aching and soreness,
gone. These were the only remedies used, and the cure
was rapid and thorough.—*J. Ferris, M. D.*

PNEUMONIA.—I gave to a case of pneumonia Ferr.
Phos., and could see the patient improving in ten minutes
after the first dose.—*Dr. H. S. Phillips.*

PNEUMONIA.—A printer, 25 years old. Found him two
days after attacked ; pulse 120 ; temperature 104.5° ; great
pain in left lung, and an unusual amount of bloody expec-
torations. Prescribed Ferr. Phos. and Kali. Mur., one
grain each every twenty minutes. Five days later, temperature 98.8°, pulse 68 ; no pain, and wanted food. No
other remedies or external applications.— *W. E. Kinnett,
M. D.*

RHEUMATISM.—All the joints of lower extremities very
much swollen, very painful with slightest movement. Severe cough ; tongue coated white ; pulse 130 ; temperature 104.5°. I gave him Mag. Phos. and Kali. Sulph. in
alternation every hour. In a short time discharged him
cured.—*Dr. J. H. Hoag.*

RHEUMATISM—ACUTE.—A young lady about 18 years
of age, bed-ridden for a week with fingers and hands badly
swollen and very tender, and feet inflamed. Pulse hard

and full, tongue white, poor appetite, restless, great weakness and disturbed sleep. I prescribed Ferr. Phos. and Kali. Mur. in alternation, and Nat. Phos. intercurrently (*i. e.*, occasionally), and Kali. Phos. at night. Two days later pains had left, swelling much less, sleep good and rapidly improving. Then she was told that it was wrong for a Christian to use medicines—should rely upon faith alone. I was called again a week later. She had relapsed, and in addition to the worse return of the former symptoms, she had a severe cough, with albuminous expectoration, and water gathering around her heart. Ordered the same treatment as before, with the addition of Nat. Mur. In twenty-four hours the gurglings about the heart had almost entirely ceased, the pains and swelling greatly improved, and she made a rapid and satisfactory recovery.—*Dr. J. B. C.*

RHEUMATISM.—A burly German lying under two blankets and a feather bed, two feet thick. Intense pain for a week from near the hip to the foot, limb numb as from paralysis. Had not slept in three nights. Ferr. Phos. 6x, and Kali. Phos. 6x, four doses in two hours and he slept. Scarcely any pain during the night. Treatment continued, and he made a quick recovery.—*J. B. Chapman, M. D.*

RHEUMATISM, INFLAMMATORY.—Mrs. S., age 72. Had not walked a step in over a year, and been treated by six different physicians. Had to be rolled on bed in sheets, and would scream at any attempt to touch her. Could not move right arm or hand, only slightly some of the fingers. I put her on Mag. Phos. and Kali Mur., 2x, and in a few months her only trouble was a little pain in stormy weather. Walks about and uses the arm as well as the other.—*G. L. Freemeyer, M. D.*

RHEUMATISM, MUSCULAR.—Dr. Schlegelman was attacked while traveling by rail, pains very severe in right side. Bryonia and electricity failed. A single dose of Ferr. Phos. cured as if by magic.

RHEUMATISM OF JOINTS—Edward B., age 12, pains in all the principal joints, but mostly in elbows and wrists, which were red and swollen, and he had some fever. Gave him Ferr. Phos. dissolved in one glass, and Kali. Mur. dissolved in another, to be taken alternately, every two hours while fever lasted, then continue Kali. Mur. alone. In a few days he was able to be out.—*Dr.*———

RHEUMATISM FROM GETTING WET.—Robert D., age 34, lives on the bank of the lake, and frequently got wet while fishing or shooting. He had pains about him for a year or two at times, sometimes in one joint and then in another. I gave him Kali. Sulph., several powders, one to be dissolved in water, a dose four times each day. In a few weeks his trouble was completely cured.—*Dr.*———

SCIATIC RHEUMATISM.—A case of sciatic rheumatism that baffled the skill of two old school physicians all winter I cured with Mag. Phos., 3x, and Ferr. Phos., 2x.—*Dr. D. Clapper.*

SCIATICA.—A lady had been suffering for two weeks with an intense pain, extending the entire length of the sciatic nerve of the left leg; slightest motion would cause cramping in leg, such as to make patient cry out. Gave powder of Ferr. Phos., 3x, and Mag. Phos., 3x. Third day patient was much better, only slight pain. On the sixth day said she never felt better in life; no pain whatever; was able to be up all the time and help about house work. I could not do without Tissue Remedies.—*D. Russell, M. D.*

SEMI-BLINDNESS, AMBLYOPIA.—Dr. F. S. McKibbon,

when 17 years old, became suddenly so nearly blind that with his best eye he could read a little with difficulty, not at all with the other. All objects were distorted and parts invisible. This continued, notwithstanding the best treatment that could be found, twenty-four years. Then Dr. T. J. Dean suggested the use of Calc. Fluor, 3x, once a day. In two months he could read with his poorest eye, and ten months later his sight was nearly perfect.—*Dr. J. B. Chapman.*

SIMULATED ANGINA PECTORIS.—Had been treated in vain for ten years by other physicians. Short, darting, spasmodic pains. Yielded at once to Mag. Phos., 6x.—*C. R. Clapp, M. D.*

SKIN TROUBLES.—Don't forget this remedy doctor, Kali. Mur., when treating skin troubles of all descriptions. I use pounds of it every year.—*Dr. Wm. Steinrauf.*

SLEEPLESSNESS.—A lady suffering with a uterine tumor had had no sleep at night for three weeks. I gave two powders of Kali. Phos., each fifteen grains, and directed her to take one at bed time, and the other in an hour, if the first did not produce sleep. She slept after the second powder, and I saw her to-day, four days later, and she says she sleeps splendidly.—*Dr.———-*

SOFT CHANCRE.—I have cured two cases of syphilis, (chancres, soft ulcerous, sloughing sores). They were as rotten cases as could well be outlined, and Kali. Mur., 2x, and Nat. Sulph., 2x, were the principal remedies, and all that was used, except in the one case that was so bad that she could not swallow anything but liquids for two days. I gave her a few doses of Kali. Iodatum, 2x. Her teeth were so loose you could have picked them out with your fingers. I suppose I would have succeeded just as well in the treatment if I had not used the Iodide, but in writing articles to go out before the profession I think we should be honest with each other, and give the truth, the whole truth, and nothing but the truth. The above mentioned cases had passed through the hands of two of the old school of our city, and now look better and made a more rapid recovery than I was ever able to do before, although I have had quite a large experience in this line for the past twenty years.—*G. L. Freemeyer, M. D.*

SORE THROAT, WITH WHITE PATCHES AND FEVER.— My little girl had a fever with sore throat and white patches in it. I gave her Kali. Mur. on going to bed at night, and the next morning she was much better, and the patches were all gone. A few doses completed the cure.—*Dr. I. L. Peebles.*

SPASMS, MUSCULAR.—Dr. A. L. Monroe says that Mag. Phos. is doing noble work for him in the treatment of the agonizing pains that accompany these spasms.

SPINAL AND STOMACH TROUBLES —Mrs. G. S., age 48. Morning frothy vomiting, excruciating· pain in stomach, headache, melancholy, sleepless, with suicidal tendencies and two very sore spots on the spine. Wished to die. Many doctors had failed to give relief. Dr. T. E. Williams put her upon Nat. Mur. in the morning, an hour later Kali. Phos. Next hour, Nat. Sulph., and so on in alternation during all waking hours. Nat. Mur. was changed to Mag. Phos. when the lightning-like pains occurred in the head. She was perfectly cured in fifteen weeks.

STOMACH.—Burning in after eating, lasting till next meal time ; tongue light gray ; no thirst, bad taste nor tenderness ; bowels regular ; sleep disturbed. Nat. Phos. cured —*Medical Era.*

STOMACH SICKNESS.—Sudden attacks of deathly sickness, coming on at no particular time, even in sleep, and lasting one-half or one hour ; appetite poor.   Ferr. Phos. cured, and appetite became ravenous.—*Dr. Rane.*

STUTTERNG.—A little girl, age four years, just recovered from convulsions, but was left with an impediment in her speech, which grew upon her.   Her mother told me it dated from the time when she had the convulsions. I gave her Mag. Phos., 3x, a small dose four times a day, and one dose of Calc. Phos., 6x, in the evening.   In three weeks she is entirely free from stuttering, except when excited or angry.   I am continuing the remedies and hope to cure completely.—*Dr.*——— ·

SUMMER COMPLAINT.—Teething children prostrated with vomiting and diarrhea, eyes half closed, inclination to roll the head, are often helped by Mag. Phos. when other remedies fail.—*Dr. Francis McMillan.*

SUNDRY DISEASES —I have used the Tissue Remedies (cell-salts) since 1874.   Have had some very severe cases of *La Grippe* this winter, but the worst have not lasted longer than one week.   One of *congestion of lungs* with hemorrhage.   Checked the hemorrhage in six hours, and the patient entirely recovered.   Another had been under allopathic treatment four weeks with constant fever. Within three days after I was called her fever left, and at the end of a week she was about the house.—*Dr. W. H. Marcan.*

Prof. Wm. Steinrauf says to his brother physicians :— Doctor, study well Nat. Mur.   In *gastric troubles* it answers a great purpose ;   indigestion with vomiting of clear, frothy water, or stringy saliva, waterbrash, water comes up the throat, longing for salt food, aversion to bread.   In *constipation* when arising from want of moisture ;   excessively dry stool producing fissure and burning pain in the rectum. In *chronic skin disease* you can't do without this remedy. In *eczema* from eating too much salt. This salt is indicated when your patient *emaciates* whilst he is living well; all exudations and secretions are transparent, slimy, like boiled staich. We often find that this medicine does good work with such *patients that are always better at the sea-shore.* When children, especially during summer complaint, have *emaciated necks.* Whenever a patient tells me, no matter what the trouble, that his or her backache is relieved by lying on something hard, this remedy is given. In *chronic rheumatism* of the joints it finds a place. In *follicular pharyngitis*, especially after our old school neighbors have been swabbing the throat with nitrate of silver, give Nat. Mur. and cure the patient without further delay. *Thrush* with much salivation, it cures. *Blisters*, like pearls around the mouth, *cracks* in the lips, *eruptions* on the chin very often call for this medicine. In *headache* it finds a prominent place. The headache is what you might call a hammering headache, generally worse in the morning. Headache of school girls. I use it very much in old *nasal and pharyngeal catarrhs* with loss of smell and taste, chronic catarrh of bloodless patients. These are but a few of the many conditions in which I have successfully used Nat. Mur. according to Schuessler.

SUPPRESSION.—Clara V., age 17 Typhoid fever two months; discharged by physician with total suppression; ankles swollen, perfectly useless and contracting muscles of knees so drawn that the joints formed right angles, and told that she would probably go into consumption. Dr. J. C. Farrell then took the case and gave Kali. Mur., 3x, every hour, and in just seven days her menses came on normally after seven months cessation. He then gave

Calc. Fluor., Calc. Phos., and Kali. Phos., and in two months she could walk ten blocks and back.

SUPPURATIONS.—Young lady, age 16.   Right foot fearfully swollen and discharging excessively.   The doctors said the foot must be amputated.   Knee joint bent at a right angle.   The mother reported the case to Dr. Schuessler, who ordered Silica once a day.   Three months later the patient walked to see the doctor with foot almost entirely healed.

Another Case.—Orphan girl, age 14.   Bone disease of foot.   Time fixed for amputation.   Dr. M. D. W. ordered Silica every hour and lotion of same on lint.   So much improvement in five days that the operation was abandoned, and in a short time she was entirely cured.

SWELLINGS.—L. P. P., face swollen as large as a goose egg on left side.   A year before had lost three weeks of time and paid his doctor $20 for treatment of a jaw injured in that place by the extraction of a tooth.   I prescribed Calc. Sulph., three or four tablets every hour, and to stop work and go home.   But he continued at work, and three days later reported, "I never saw the like of that in my life.   I continued work, but took the medicine every hour, and before 10 o'clock the swelling was going down, and the next morning it was all gone.—*Dr. H. S. Phillips.*

SYPHILIS.—Laay, aged 50, with syphilitic ulcers on back and lower half of right leg.   The left leg had had ulcers all around it just above the ankle.   At this time it had one so deep that splinters of bone have been discharged, and another on which the flesh was hanging loose.   The odor was something dreadful.   Had suffered a hundred deaths with them.   Been treated by every doctor in the county.   Could not lie down, and could not sleep, except propped up with pillows.   I gave Kali. Phos.,

Ferr. Phos. and Silica for two weeks, when she could lie down and sleep. I then added Calc. Sulph. three times daily. The ulcers on back and right leg are now entirely cured. The flesh on the left leg has become firm and one ulcer healed, and she is well in every way except the re-- maining ulcer. Will report as to it. To one and all I would say, Try the "Twelve Manner of Fruits" (cell-salts) for the "Healing of the Nations."—*Dr. Wm. Mc-Innes.*

TAPE-WORM.—A boy, age five years, had spasm, and been treated by several physicians without benefit. After using Nat. Phos. 3x, for six weeks three times a day, he passed four feet three inches of tape-worm, much to the astonishment of all interested. It is believed the entire worm passed, as there was no evidence of any remaining. Nat. Phos. is especially efficient in cases of pin-worms.—*Dr. A. C. Kimball.*

TAPE-WORM.—The characteristics of this case were: Great lassitude in forenoons, very sleepy in the early part of the night, sleep soundly until 4 A. M., when he would be awakened by keen-cutting pain in the bowels and diarrhœa, which would keep up for about three hours, and end in extreme prostration. After eating a little breakfast diarrhœa would cease, and patient would feel better until late in the afternoon, when he would be the same as in the morning. This kept up with great regularity until Nat. Phos., 3x, was taken. The next seance brought with it results in the shape of a twenty-six foot tape-worm, and the commingled emotions of surprise, disgust, and satisfaction of the patient, who had been unable up to that time to diagnose his case. Recovery was rapid — *Dr. N. O. Brenizer.*

TEETHING.—Child, 18 months old, had cut but two

lower lateral incisors, and the molars of lower and upper jaw. Thin, poorly nourished, "pigeon-breast" chest; hard to learn to walk, general lack of osseous development. Gave Calc. Phos., 3x, three times a day, thirty powders, corrected nourishment. Did not see the case again in three months, when I hardly recognized my scrawny patient, now a strong, healthy child. Had all the incisors, the molars and the " stomach." teeth were beginning to show. Continued treatment as before.

TEETHING —Child, 18 months old; hot skin; cheeks highly flushed; sparkling eyes; pupils dilated, and extreme restlessness and irritability. Ferr. Phos., 6x trit., in water every hour. The first dose had a decided quieting effect, the child going to sleep shortly after taking it, and the cheeks becoming much less flushed. A few repetitions of the remedy entirely removed all the dental irritation.—*Dr. Wilde.*

TOOTHACHE, ODONTALGIA.—Lady, face fearfully swollen, no sleep for two nights, great pain. Ordered one grain of Mag. Phos. every half hour. Pain gone in two hours, and the swelling soon subsided.— *W. E. Kinnett, M. D.*

TOOTHACHE.—A young married lady, severe neuralgia and toothache for several days. Cocaine, morphine and other drugs had all failed, and she was almost crazy with the pain. I gave Mag. Phos. and hot fomentations, but she grew worse. Calc. Phos. gave no better results. I then asked her to try cold water on the tooth, and finding that it mitigated the pain I gave Ferr. Phos. for inflamed nerve, and in half an hour she was asleep, and by continuing the remedy she recovered.—*J. B. Chapman, M. D.*

TRANSMITTED DISEASE.—A little girl of three years,

with glands of neck swollen to the size of a hen's egg. Also glands under the arms and in the groins were greatly swollen, and had been more than a year Pale, anæmic, had cut teeth slowly, very constipated. Her mother when pregnant, had incipient consumption, but when the child was born, she was left healthy and strong. I prescribed Calc. Phos. and Silica, and occasionally Calc. Fluor, for the hardness of the glands, and after several months, she was perfectly cured.—*J B. Chapman, M. D.*

TYPHLITIS (Inflammation of the coecum and vermiform appendix).—Charles M., age 18, found in bed suffering intense pain and vomiting large quantities of greenish substance ; pulse 125, with a temperature of 104 F. I found a large tumory swelling situated in the right illiac fossa. It was of a deep, reddish, inflammatory hue, and so tender and sensitive that the patient would hardly allow me to touch the parts. My diagnosis was typhlitis, and well advanced at that. Vomiting was persistent. I placed in a glass two-thirds full of water thirty grains of Nat. Sulph., 3x, and ordered to be given one teaspoonful of the solution until vomiting would be arrested, which took place at 10 P. M., or nine hours after I first saw the patient. I now discontinued Nat. Sulph., and placed the patient on Ferr. Phos. and Kali. Mur., thirty grains of each, dissolved in two separate glasses, two-thirds full of water ; gave one teaspoonful alternately every hour. In a few days the swelling began to disappear. The medicine not given as often as before. His recovery in the end was good.—*Dr. T E. Williams.*

ULCERATED SORE THROAT.—Symptoms high fever, rapid pulse, pain all over, sore throat with swollen tonsils, and deep, ragged, white ulcers, and very offensive breath. I gave Ferr. Phos. for the fever and inflammatory conditions; Kali. Mur for white tongue and ulcers, and a gargle of the same used frequently. This has been sufficient in all cases to insure a quick recovery.—*Dr. J. B. Chapman.*

ULCERATED TOOTH AND GUM BOIL.—Lillie, 6 years old. I gave her about forty doses of Calc. Sulph., 3x, which should have lasted her ten days or more; but she took them all in three days, and was perfectly cured in that time.—*M. F. Richards, M. D.*

URINATION, FREQUENT AND PAINFUL.—In women, the attacks coming on suddenly, constant urging, with little relief, of nervous origin; I have used Mag. Phos., with most satisfactory results.—*Dr. Frances McMillan.*

URINE, SUPPRESSION OF.—A man 100 years old, that came under my care. This man had been sixty hours without any water passage. He had taken during the time about six ounces of Nitre, besides a large quantity of melon-seed and cuckleburr tea.

When I was called I used the catheter and drew off a little more than one pint of blood. The next morning I drew off another pint of pure blood. I gave remedies to control the hemorrhage from the kidneys, but it did not stop it. The same day, at night, I drew off another pint. There was also a spasmodic contraction of the neck of the bladder, which I knew would have to be overcome before he could pass anything. The next morning I drew off another pint, making two quarts in all. I prescribed Ferr. Phos., 3x, about four grains in a cupful of water. Of this I directed a teaspoonful every hour. I visited him again at night and the bleeding had all stopped. He was able to pass a few drops of urine. I then changed to Mag. Phos., 3x, and the next morning he could pass water quite freely. Then inflammation of the small intestines set in with watery vomiting. , The bowels were swollen very much, and were very tender. Constipation was present, with loss of appetite. I commenced the use of Nat. Mur., 3x, and Kali. Phos . 3x, in alternation every hour. Twelve hours sufficed to control that trouble, and to finish up the case I put him on Kali. Mur., 3x. every two hours. I consider this a remarkable case in view of the age.—*Dr. A. K.*

URINE, INCONTINENCE OF.—Mrs. M., age 34, suffered from incontinence of urine for three years; origin unknown. Ferr. Phos., 6x, four times a day gave relief in a week, and cured in four weeks.—*Dr.* ———

CHAPTER III.

THE BIOCHEMIC SYSTEM EXPLAINED.

In order to an adequate comprehension of this system of cure, we must know—

1. WHAT DISEASE ("NOT AT EASE") IS.

To disabuse the mind of the reader of the life-long notion that disease is some entity to be expelled or to be killed, is one of the most difficult tasks of Biochemic teachers.

In order to make the subject plain we will premise that there are two, and only two classes of disease. The first is primary, the other secondary. The primary consists of those departures from health which are the immediate result of the lack of a sufficient supply of the organic blood foods, i. e., albumen, sugar and fat, or of the inorganic blood foods, i. e., the twelve cell-salts, or of water or of oxygen.

The lack of any one of these seventeen elements of organic life, to the extent that that deficiency interferes with and prevents its proper function in the animal body, is *primary disease*.

The one chief characteristic of all primary disease (by whatever name it may be called in medical books) is that it is *curable* simply by the supply of the deficient element.

The next important characteristic of all primary disease is that it is always liable by bacterial germination or inoculation to become secondary.

The chief characteristic of secondary disease is, its curability depends upon the two-fold process of *supply* of the *deficient element* and the *destruction* of the *bacterial inva-*

ders by *germicides* in all cases in which the white blood corpuscles (which are the physiological germicides) are unable to annihilate them.

The objection may be made, that according to this statement hunger and thirst are primary diseases.

The answer is, So they are the instant they reach the extent of disturbance of the functions which food and drink normally sustain. Up to that point they are simply nature's signals for relief before damage is inflicted.

It is very questionable whether there are any diseases that are not first primary and easily curable in that stage, for science has demonstrated that the leucocytes (white blood corpuscles) of perfectly healthy blood have the power to overmaster all forms of bacterial invasion.

Pure blood is that which contains the twelve mineral constituents in the right proportion. MICROBES CANNOT LIVE IN SUCH BLOOD.

The question arises here, naturally, why should deficiency of these salts ever occur? Answer: A failure to procure a sufficient amount of the proper kinds of food cuts the supply of cell salts off at the fountain, or if disease already exists, poor digestion or assimilation may waste even an adequate supply in the food. Again, some great excess of heat or cold, or some sudden and severe electrical change may make an unusual demand upon the blood and partially exhaust its supply too rapidly to be immediately restored by the food. So locally the circulation may be mechanically obstructed and thus have the same effect as if the food were inefficient, or as if digestion and assimilation were defective. Likewise cold, heat, overwork (mental or physical) or exhausting electrical changes may, in a limited area, produce the same result that an overdrain upon the blood does generally.

It is with cell life just as it is with water drops turning a wheel, each drop does its work in passing over the wheel then is gone, becomes dead to it, and other drops follow, and·the wheel continues to turn by the constant succession of the drops. Suppose that the molecular movements of the water are so changed that it becomes steam, then disturbance occurs at once in the motion of the wheel because it is not adapted to the new form of molecular motion, and is out of harmony with the motive power.

So disease is molecular motion of the cell salts out of harmony with the motive power, i. e., the life force, because of a diminished quantity of one or more of the cell salts.

It would be just as sensible to sledge off the flanges or buckets of the wheel to cure it, as it is to introduce into the human system agents that do violence to its organism.

All that the wheel wants is water instead of steam. All that the body wants is enough of the cell salts to change their molecular motions into harmony with the life force and evolve new cells according to its own type of creation instead of a lower.

Disease is not therefore an entity, a poison, a something to be killed or expelled by the use of dangerous substances supposed to have an innate hostility to it, in the interests of humanity ; it is simply a privation. It is true that after a time chemical products may be formed from the defective vital processes that may have a very positive and harmful effect, but these are results of disease, not disease itself.

Then if effects need attention let them be antidoted upon precisely the same principles that the chemist does in his laboratory, always bearing in mind the different conditions which vitality imposes.

" We no longer should dose man as a *whole* to cure him,

'but we should strive to interpret the nature of the cells forming his tissues, their activities, their reactions to drugs and physical treatment, and we should minister to these microscopic individuals or aggregations with a view to increase their natural functions in the prevention of disease, or create activities of this character."—*Dr. Paul Paquin.*

There are but twelve primary abnormal conditions, though they may be called by a thousand names, and these twelve conditions are cured by the twelve cell salts.

2. WHAT THE CELL-SALTS ARE.

If an animal body be burned, the ash that remains is its indestructible mineral elements.

These are eight in number, viz: Potassa, soda, lime, magnesia, iron, fluorine, sulphur and silica. But in the body—

The *lime* combines with phosphorus, sulphur and fluorine, into three compounds, viz:

Calcarea Phosphorica=Calcium Phosphate, i. e., Phosphate of lime. Cell-Salt abbreviation, Calc. Phos.

Calcarea Sulphorica=Calcium Sulphate, i. e., Gypsum, Plaster of Paris. Cell-Salt abbreviation, Calc. Sulph.

Calcarea Fluorica=Calcium Fluoride, i. e., Fluoride of lime, Fluor. Spar. Cell-Salt abbreviation, Calc. Fluor.

The *potassa* combines with phosphorus, sulphur and muriatic acid, into three compounds, viz:

Kali. Phosphoricum=Potassium Phosphate, i. e., Phosphate of potash. Cell-Salt abbreviation, Kali. Phos.

Kali. Sulphuricum=Potassium sulphate, i. e., Sulphate of potash. Cell-Salt abbreviation, Kali. Sulph.

Kali. Muriaticum=Potassium chloride, i. e., Chloride of potash. Cell-Salt abbreviation, Kali. Mur.

The *soda* combines with muriatic acid, phosphorus and sulphur into three compounds, viz:

Natrum Phosphoricum=Sodium phosphate, i. e., Phosphate of soda.   Cell-Salt abbreviation, Nat. Phos.

Natrum Muriaticum=Sodium Choride, i. e., common salt.   Cell-Salt abbreviation, Nat. Mur.

Natrum Sulphurica=Sodium sulphate, i. e., Glauber's salt, sulphate of soda. Cell-Salt abbreviation, Nat. Sulph.

The *magnesia* combines with phosphorus into one compound, viz:

Magnesia Phosphorica=Magnesium phosphate, i. e., Phosphate of magnesia.   Cell-Salt abbreviation, Mag. Phos.

The *iron* combines with phosphorus into one compound, viz:

Ferrum Phosphoricum=Ferri phosphas, i. e., Phosphate of iron.   Cell-Salt abbreviation, Ferr. Phos.

The *silica* remains uncombined.

Silica, i. e., Silicious earth, pure flint or quartz. Cell-Salt abbreviation, Silica.

Therefore the Cell-Salts (mode of preparation of which will be explained a little further on) are to supply the deficiencies of these compounds, not merely of their eight mineral bases.

These always exists in certain definite proportions in healthy human blood; therefore they are natural and friendly to the system, while the remedies of all other schools are unfriendly to the body, and it is the effort of nature to expel them that produces their physiological action.

3. THE PHYSIOLOGICAL PROPERTIES OF THE CELL-SALTS, AND THEIR PARTICULAR FUNCTIONS.

As employed in Biochemic practice, unlike most drug

medicines, they are neither very sweet nor sour, nor bitter, cathartic, diuretic, nor stimulating, but summed up in a single sentence, their properties are *assimilative* of the organic elements, sugar, fat and albumen.

The body and all its fluids are made of the Cell-Salts and water as inorganic constituents, in combination with the three organic compounds, sugar, fat and albumen.

But, though these may be in close juxtaposition, there can be no body-building without the mysterious life-force to originate and guide the process. This life-force acts upon the Cell-Salts, producing vital molecular movements in them, depending in character upon the quantity of the Salt acted upon, just as a certain number of vibrations of light produce yellow and another number shows as red.

These vital molecular movements reveal themselves as affinities for organic substances. Each Salt has its own particular affinity, one for fat, another for sugar, another for albumen. These affinities thus set in play by the life-force, effect a chemico-vital union of each Salt with its appropriate organic mate, thus forming the cells, which are the base of all animal structures, and the aggregations of which cells make tissue—bone tissue, fat tissue, etc., according to the nature of the Salt employed as the primary worker.

If the quantity of a particular Salt be not sufficient to accomplish the purpose of the life-force, cell-evolution will go on notwithstanding, but on a lower plane, therefore abnormal, because its lower type of organization unfits it to perform the functions of the higher.

The functions of the Cell-Salts may be stated more specifically thus:

CALC. PHOS. unites with albumen for the replenishment of connective (glue forming) tissues, blood corpuscles and the gastric juice, and also particularly of the bones, which consist of the lime which this Salt provides to the extent of 57 per cent. of their substance.

In normal proportions it preserves against anæmia, re-pairs fractures, secures normal teething, and to some extent supplies deficiencies of Mag. Phos.

When deficient it permits the easily decomposing albu-men to act as a foreign substance in the blood, and be expelled in the expectoration as mucus discharges, or as albumen from the kidneys. or as pimples, or eczema of the skin, or as scrofula. It also causes indigestion ; head-ache with cold feeling in the head ; thinness and softness of the skull, delayed closing or reopening of its fonta-nells (seams) ; dropsy of the brain ; aching eyeballs ; nasal polypi ; cold in head with thick, tough discharge ; rheu-matism ; various teething disorders ; chronic enlargement of the tonsils ; constant hoarseness ; vomiting after cold drink ; prolapsus ; cough, with expectoration of albumi-nous, white mucus ; curvature of the spine ; numb, cold limbs ; bow-legs ; bone abscesses ; paralysis with creep-ing numbness and coldness ; rickets ; night sweats in con-sumptions, etc.

Its chief characteristics are: Worse by cold, motion, change of weather and getting wet; better by rest, warmth and lying down.

CALC. SULPH. carries waste matters from the system by the organs of excretion, i. e., skin, lungs, kidneys and bowels.

When in normal proportion it restrains suppurative pro-cesses and heals suppurations by removing their exciting causes.

When deficient, it permits the epithelial cells to disinte-grate and with the wastes to be cast out as discharges or suppurations of a yellow, purulent character, or as crusts of the same, as in the third stages of all catarrhs, lung troubles, boils, carbuncles, ulcers or abscesses; suppurations of the head, eyes, ears, nose; watery pimples on face; ulcers of teeth, mouth, tongue, throat; diarrhea, dysentery with pus-like discharges; chronic inflammation of bladder; suppuration of the breast or joints; all wounds in the suppurative stage; all cases of suppuration when the discharges continue too long and the sore is unhealthy.

Its chief characteristics are: Worse by getting wet, or by washing or working in water; also, the discharge of pus with an open vent.

CALC. FLUOR. builds the elastic fiber of the muscles, skin, connective (glue-forming) tissue and walls of the blood vessels out of albumen, water and oxygen. (Albumen is a compound of protein, sulphur and phosphorus. Protein is a compound of nitrogen, carbon, hydrogen and oxygen).

Calc. Fluor. also controls the formation of the surface of bones and the enamel of teeth.

In normal proportions it therefore preserves the elastic fibers intact, and in concert with Ferr. Phos. as an element of tonicity, secures their vigorous action.

When deficient, the elastic fibers sag, and varicose veins, vascular tumors, hemorrhoids (piles), prolapsus, etc., occur; or if an elastic fiber or lime exudation finds place in the connective tissue or the glandular system, it cannot be absorbed because of the deficient action of the minute blood vessels and swelling supervenes.

Its deficiency also gives an unhealthy condition to the surface of the bones and the enamel of the teeth; also causes tumors on the heads of young infants; cataract of the eye ; diseases of the bones of the ear, or of the nose, or jaw ; also stuffy cold in the head with thick, yellow, lumpish, greenish discharge ; also makes the teeth very brittle, or loose in their sockets, or the enamel rough ; also gives cracked tongue ; elongation of palate ; piles ; displacements ; coughs with tiny lumps of tough yellow mucus ; varicose veins ; chapped skin ; skin hard and horny ; hard swellings ; dropsy from heart disease, etc.

Its chief characteristics are: Worse in damp weather, better generally by hot applications in hardened conditions, and by cold when contraction is required; also relieved by fomentation and by rubbing. It is complementary with Silica; should be used when Silica is indicated, but fails to complete the cure.

FERR. PHOS. is a constituent of the blood corpuscles for the double purpose of furnishing iron to the muscle-cells and of carrying oxygen to those cells.

When in normal proportions it preserves the tone of the circular fibers of the blood vessels, and thus prevents varicose veins and hemorrhage ; preserves the muscles of the intestinal villi (absorbents) from relaxation and consequent loose evacuations ; prevents the muscles of the intestinal walls from weakening, thereby causing their vermicular (worm-like) action to diminish and constipation to set in ; gives contractility to the blood vessels that are overcharged in congestions, so that the irritation is removed ; and furnishes oxygen for the reconstructive process of cell building, whether of the healing of fresh wounds or replacement of worn out tissue.

When deficient, the circulation increases in the effort to make the part do the oxygen carrying work of the whole, which more rapid circulation generates too much heat (fever) which causes a deficiency in potassium chloride, and as this salt works with fibrin, that cannot all be built into tissues, consequently remains as a foreign agent in the blood to be thrown off through the lungs by expectoration, or remaining in the lung inflames it into pneumonia, or is expelled through the nasal membrane as catarrh (Carey); also causes rush of blood to the head, headache, vertigo; inflammation of the eyes, ears, mouth, tongue, throat, stomach, lungs, bladder and other pelvic organs; and hemorrhage of bright red blood, anaemia, etc.

Its chief characteristics are: Always aggravated by motion and relieved by cold.

KALI. MUR. finds in the blood certain albuminoids (nitrogenous substances) with which it unites and forms fibrine (blood-clot). (Carey).

Its function therefore is to change the nitrogenous element of food into flesh, because fibrine is flesh as yet in a liquid medium.

Prof. Stockois, at the last Medical Congress, at Rome, declared that " It can be chemically demonstrated that Kali. Mur. can both bind two atoms of oxygen and form ozone, and under different conditions of the system it can break up the ozone and thus make two atoms of oxygen available for the processes of life." What is this but practical storage of oxygen for emergencies?

In normal proportions it preserves muscular weight and vigor.

When deficient, the unused fibrinous elements are cast out in the form of fibrinous exudations, such as the false membranes of croups, diphtheria and dysentery, and the serous exudations containing fibrine in acute inflammations of the pleura and peritoneum, and in the thick white discharges from mucus membranes, and in the white contents of skin eruptions and the flour-like scales on the skin.

The same material, failing to be organized into tissues, causes soft infiltrations (swellings), headaches with thick white coating on tongue; thick white discharges from the eyes, ears, nose; cankered mouth; gum-boils; ulcerated sore throat; gastritis (inflammation of stomach), second stage; sluggish liver, with constipation; diarrhea, with pale yellow or gray-colored stools; all thick, milky white, non-irritating mucus discharges; rheumatism with swelling; chronic swelling of feet and legs; epilepsy; blistering erysipelas: glandular swellings, etc.

Its chief characteristics are: Generally worse from motion; if in stomach or abdomen worse from pastry, rich or fatty foods; also from a highly albuminous diet.

KALI. PHOS. makes the gray matter of the brain out of albumen, sugar, oil, water and oxygen. It is also a constituent of the brain, the nerves, the muscles and the blood-corpuscles.

Existing in normal proportions it maintains mental and nervous strength, and properly innervates (i. e., supplies with nerve strength) all parts of the organism.

When deficient it may cause any disease that will naturally result from deficiency of brain and nerve power; and of course aggravate all diseases caused by the lack of other Cell-Salts. The range of its action, therefore, is almost universal.

Its chief characteristics are: Worse by noise, by rising from a sitting position; by mental or physical exertion, and in cold air. Better by gentle motion, eating, excitement, or any gentle, pleasing, mental occupation.

KALI. SULPH. carries organic matter—i. e., oil, sugar and albumen, especially oil—to the cells of the skin and mucous membranes, and thus vitalizes the tissues of the pores.

When in normal proportions it keeps open the 7,000,-000 pores of the skin, which are constantly throwing off the wastes of the system.

When deficient, the skin not receiving a proper amount of oil, the pores schrivel, the excretion of waste matters through them is suppressed, and the blood thereby becomes poisoned.

Its chief characteristics are: Worse in warm room and toward evening; better in cool, open air; yellow mucous discharges; always applicable in third stage of inflammation.

MAG. PHOS. forms out of water, albumen and oxygen, the transparent fluid that nourishes and governs the delicate nerve-threads called white fibers.

In normal proportions it preserves muscular tissues from undue or spasmodic contraction.

As compared with Kali. Phos., the function of which is to supply the stimulus for contraction, Mag. Phos. acts as a regulator.

When deficient, spasmodic action is set up in the form of cramps, jerks, and spasmodic pains.

As compared with Ferrum Phos., a deficiency of which produces muscular relaxation, the deficiency of Mag. Phos. produces undue contractility, hence come twitchings, lockjaw, convulsions, choking on attempt to swallow, squinting, sharp neuralgic pains, spasmodic stammering, griping, indigestion, painful urination, dysmenorrhea, convulsive coughing, nervous chills with chattering teeth, yawning with straining of lower jaw, etc., which are all Nature's cry for more Mag. Phos.

Its chief characteristics are, as an antispasmodic: Worse

on right side from cold, cold air, washing in cold water and from touch.   Better by warmth, pressure, friction and bending double.

NAT. MUR. distributes water in right proportions to all parts of the system.   About 70 per cent. of our bodies consists of water, which would be distributed only in obedience to the laws of gravitation, the propulsion of the circulation and the permeability of tissues by fluids, were it not for Nat. Mur.   This Salt uses the water both to build up tissue and to carry off wastes, and as these double processes go on continuously in every part, its importance can scarcely be overestimated.

In normal proportions it gives to all the excretions and secretions a proper degree of moisture or fluidity, and maintains the same in all the structures.

When deficient, there will be a decrease of secretions, or greater dryness of excretions, or two little water in the tissues ; as in sunstroke drying the base of the brain ; delirium tremens drying the brain substance ; delirium with tongue either frothy or dry and parched ; headaches ; melancholia, hopelessness, despondence with constipation and watery symptoms elsewhere ; loss of smell from dryness of the nose ; low fevers with dryness of tongue ; constipation with dry stools ; dry coughs and dry skin.

On the other hand, the deficiency of Nat. Mur. may occasion increase of secretions, e. g., saliva or tears, or an increase of water in the tissues, e. g., dropsy ; also neuralgic pains in eyes ; fresh colds, with free discharge of water from the nostrils ; vomiting of clear mucus ; salivation ; catarrhs with transparent watery discharge ; diarrhea with watery stools ; excessive urination ; asthma ; bronchitis with frothy, watery mucus ; palpitation of the heart with dropsical swellings ; watery skin eruptions ; excessive sleep from too much moisture in the brain, etc.

Its chief characteristics are: Worse in morning, cold weather and salty air; better in evening.

NAT. PHOS. splits up the lactic acid formed in the process of digestion into carbonic acid and water ; also combines with acid into new compounds. The importance of this salt is shown by the fact stated by Bernard, that a very weak solution of acetic or lactic acid injected directly into the blood will cause death even before it is neutralized by the alkali in the blood.

In normal proportions it gives the alkaline quality to blood and saliva by neutralizing the excess of acid that would otherwise exist from the fact that the creation of acid is an organic process and is never deficient, if a sufficient amount of proper food is taken.

When deficient, it causes all diseases that spring from excess of acidity, e. g., inflammation of eyes with creamy discharge ; acidity of the stomach ; sore throat with creamy coating ; false diphtheria ; morning sickness with vomiting of sour fluid ; ulceration of stomach with creamy yellow coating on tongue ; diarrhea with green, sour smelling stools ; inability to retain urine ; trembling about the heart after eating ; rheumatic pains with sour smelling perspiration : skin diseases with creamy yellow secretion ; diabetes, etc.

Characteristic indications are: A moist, thick, golden-yellow coating on the tongue and palate, and acidity.

NAT. SULPH. eliminates excess of water from the blood and tissues, and preserves the bile in normal consistency.

In normal proportions it prevents the accumulation in the tissues of the water that is formed by their constant oxydation ; also prevents excessive accumulation in the blood of the water that is held in solution by the air of respiration ; also prevents the accumulation in the digestive tract of the water formed by the decomposition of lactic acid. (Carey).

When deficient, excess of water accumulates in the blood and causes chills ; the bile thickens, clogs the ducts, and produces biliousness, vertigo, yellow eyes and skin ; bad taste in mouth ; dirty greenish gray or greenish brown tongue, or a white or gray coated tongue ; diarrhea with dark greenish stools ; diabetes ; brick dust urine ; rheumatism with bilious symptoms ; lassitude ; consumption with yellow watery and green expectoration, etc.

As related to Natrum Mur., which carries water into and distributes it in proper quantities through the system, Nat. Sulph. carries it out of the tissues into the excretory channels.

Its chief characteristics are: Worse by use of water in any form, in damp weather, in the morning, and by lying on left side; better in warm, dry weather, and in open air.

SILICA mechanically promotes suppuration by the lancet-like action of its infinitesimal crystals, and is an electrical conductor for the gray matter of the brain. (Carey). It is a component part of the connective tissue, the epidermis, the hair and the nails.

In normal proportions it affects the brain, spinal marrow and nerves favorably through the connective tissue covering of the nerve fibers.

When deficient, it causes swelling of the connective tissue cells which may go on to suppuration, as in boils, felons, carbuncles, suppuration of glands, joints, cornea ot the eye, and the like. It may also render the connective tissue of the brain so negative that thought becomes difficult and despondency or headache supervene, etc.

Its chief characteristics are: `Worse at night, during full moon, from chilling feet and in open air; better by heat and in warm room.*

An important fact to be noted just here is the COMPEN-SATIVE FUNCTION of these salts, i. e., by reason of their chemical affinities if one salt becomes deficient, it may be reinforced by drawing upon another that is chemically related to it, e. g., when excess of brain work or worry has reduced the supply of Kali. Phos. it may be measurably substitutionally provided by the other phosphate salts, viz., Calc. Phos., Mag. Phos. and Nat. Phos.; but that supply is inferior for the use of the brain, besides exhausting the stock of the substituted salt to such an extent as to interfere with its appropriate work.

This explains how, by a sort of patch-work compensation, one can live for many years notwithstanding the presence of what would otherwise be a fatal deficiency in a particular salt, yet never really recover health, because Nature's effort to run the machine in spite of the defect entails other deficiencies that in turn may find other substitutions, and so on, until nearly every salt has become insufficient.

This also explains why the supply of the chief deficiency only so often fails to cure, i. e., because the other needs are not met. A balloon may have one main leak and five smaller ones, all of which together render it impossible to expand it, because they let off the gas as fast as it can be supplied.

The largest leak may then be stopped, but still complete expansion can never be had and a safe ascent secured until all the other five are mended. So with the Cell-Salts. If one is at hard work, as well try to sustain the energies of the system by eating sugar alone, as to keep up the normal health upon one or even *eleven* of these necessary elements of organic life ; the machine is designed to work perfectly on *twelve*, and *all* of them must be provided, for Nature cannot be defrauded with impunity, nor can she work her best on any other plan than her chosen one.

The importance of the separate functions of the several salts will be fully seen when their use in the cure of disease comes to be considered.

4. HOW THE CELL-SALTS CURE DISEASE.

Simply by supplying the lack.

The fever-pangs of excessive thirst need only water to be assuaged.

The agonies of starvation require only rest and food to be subdued.

The obtuse mentality and sluggish action of the vital organs in deficient oxydation call only for that life-inspiring element.

So, whatever the particular phase of primary disease may be, resulting from a deficiency of a single Cell-Salt, the one only call that its symptoms make, is for the inorganic food for the lack of which the blood is starving.

For example : Kali. Sulph. has been deficient until an eczema with dry itching skin is telling that the skin lacks its proper nourishment.

To other schools of medicine that voice calls for nerve-quieting unguents and bacterial destroyers. If these remedies chance to contain the element for lack of which the skin is suffering, they may cure by virtue of that element ; but most likely they do not, and the disease goes on.

To the Biochemist that voice simply says, "Give me Kali. Sulph." ; and it is done ; and if the disease is yet in its primary stage, its vitalizing influence *cures at once.* If it has reached the secondary stage, he must run the same chance of selecting the right germicide that others do, with still this great advantage in his favor: he supplies the need for nutriment at the same time that he seeks to destroy the germs which perpetuate the trouble.

Take another illustration: Kali. Mur. is deficient: because of it, the albuminous element in the blood which should be made into fibrine (lean flesh) cannot be, because it is the special function of Kali. Mur. to effect that transformation. The albumen is chemically too unstable to go floating long in the moist, warm blood-current without putrefaction; therefore, as soon as it fails to be built into tissue it becomes a source of peril, hence wise Nature seeks to cast it forth as waste material before it can do serious damage.

If there is not oxygen enough to change it into urea and expel it through the kidneys, or if there is a local irritation of the throat determining the blood to that locality, Nature will cast it off through the mucous membrane as an exudation which by infection may become almost instantly croup or diphtheria.

Supply the needed Salt and the albumen in the blood is at once assimilated, and of necessity the exudation must cease for want of material.

The seeming mystery of cures by such simple means should now be explained.

Science has shown that the nearer the primary atomic form of matter any substance can be found, the more it becomes capable of penetrating other bodies. Hence the ether that fills space, as undoubtedly the nearest to atomic existence of any known substance, has a penetrating power that nothing can resist as proved by the recent discovery of the telegraphic ray, so much more potent than the X-ray.

The crude Salts are always in molecular, i. e., aggregated form.

The more they are triturated, the more they approach, though probably they never reach the atomic condition.

It is therefore perfectly clear that triturations or dilutions from triturations are the only proper form for remedial use.

Trituration consists in rubbing a Cell-Salt in a mortar not less than one to six hours with nine times its weight of sugar of milk, which is selected to be the vehicle for the administration of the Salt, because it is harmless, pleasant to the taste, occasions no chemical change in any of the Salts, and is itself an element of the living organism.

This makes the first trituration or potency, and is expressed by the sign, if any be used, 1x.

The second trituration or potency (the words mean the same thing as far as relative proportions of the Salt and its vehicle go, but trituration is confined exclusively to the powder or tablet form, while potency applies to liquids and powders) is made, not by mixing one part of the mineral Salt directly with 99 parts of the sugar of milk but by taking one part of the 1x and rubbing that with 99 parts of the sugar of milk one to six hours more.

The difference in effect is very great. If the Salt were used by direct mixture for the second potency (trituration, 2x), then it would have but the same degree of comminution or breaking up into greater fineness as the 1x, whereas by taking the one part of the 1x of which to make the 2x, it undergoes double the amount of friction.

The rapid diminution of the relative proportion of the

. mineral salt to that of its vehicle (sugar of milk) is seen by this statement, viz., the 1x is salt one-tenth grain to sugar of milk nine-tenths of a grain.

The 2x = salt 1-100 of a grain to 99-100 of its vehicle.

The 3x = salt 1-1,000 of a grain to 999-1,000 of its vehicle.

The 4x = salt 1-10,000 of a grain to 9,999-10,000 of its vehicle.

The 5x = salt 1-100,000 of a grain to 99,999-100,000 of its vehicle.

The 6x = salt 1-1,000,000 of a grain to 999,999-1,000,000 of its vehicle.

The 7x = salt 1-10,000,000 of a grain to 9,999,999-10,000,000 of its vehicle.

The 8x = salt 1-100,000,000 of a grain to 99,999,999-100,000,000 of its vehicle.

The 9x = salt 1-1,000,000,000 of a grain to 999,999,999-1,000,000,000 of its vehicle.

The 10x = salt 1-10,000,000,000 of a grain to 9,999,999,999-10,000,000,000 of its vehicle, and so on to the desired potency, if any higher be deemed advisable.

The thought naturally arises, how can such infinitesimal quantities of any food such as is represented by the 6x have any effect whatever upon the vital processes?

The answer may be found in the following facts, viz:

Scientists estimate that one milligramme (i. e., the thousandth part of a French gramme, which gramme equals 15.438 grains troy, the 1-1,000 part of which is .0154 of one troy grain) of any substance contains sixteen trillions (16,000,000,000,000 French; the English would be 16,-000,000,000,000,000,000) of the ultimate molecules of that substance, or 2,464,000,000,000,000 molecules to each troy grain.

The 6x salt contains in one grain one-millionth of a grain of the salt, i. e., 2,464,000,000 of its atoms. As the · dose consists of three grains, there are therefore in each dose of the 6x, 7,392,000,000 atoms—a respectable number certainly.

But this alone does not meet the question. We must know also, at least to a reasonable degree of probability, how many atoms are requisite to supply deficiency. This in turn must depend upon the amount of the deficiency.

This raises the question of dosage.

It would add greatly to exact knowledge concerning it if we could know precisely the line of demarkation between the physiological hunger for a deficient salt, and the pathological disease indications that the hunger has not been satisfied. It is altogether probable that a certain definite percentage of waste beyond supply *is that line*, but experiments have never settled it, even if they have been attempted.

Knowing the quantity of the salt, and assuming a proportionate waste, if we knew the percentage which makes the line between salt-hunger and disease from lack of the salt, we could calculate accurately the amount to be supplied, and the dosage would then be very simple.

In our ignorance of that we can only show by a mathematical process the certainty of being able to supply all probable deficiency.

On the fair assumption that the infant appropriates all the iron each day that its one quart of milk food contains, i. e., one milligram to each half pint, there are supplied to its 4,115 drops of blood each day 8,333,333,333 molecules of iron or 347,222,222 each hour, which is 86,809 atoms to every drop of blood, or 357,219,035 atoms at any one hour.   The same milk contains but one-billionth of a grain of fluorine, while of the iron there is six-millionths of a grain.

It is fair to assume that the reduction in ordinary food from the working to the bare subsistence standpoint represents all the privation that the system can endure without detriment. This is 48 per cent. Anything below must be disease-producing. This per cent is equivalent to the loss of 171,466,136 atoms, which would be supplied by one-forty-second part of a three-grain dose of the Ferrum Phos.

Now if the loss in any disease be even forty-two times greater than the diminution from the work to the subsistence standpoint, even then a single three-grain dose would supply the deficiency. This proves conclusively that the infinitesimal quantities of the 6x are abundant to supply the losses which produce disease.

As further illustrations of the power of infinitesimals:

The one-thouasndth part of a grain of strychnia will produce tetanus in frogs.—*Dr. Arnold, of Heidelberg.*

He has seen this result repeatedly from one-millionth of a grain.—*Hygieia, Vol. X, p. 56.*

Professor Stokvis, in an address given at the Medical Congress in Rome, made use of the following example: "If we throw metallic copper into water and wait for some days, we shall find that a certain proportion of the copper has dissolved, i. e., one part to seventy-seven million parts of water" (about one drop to three barrels of water), and Dr. Walker adds: "Drinking such water may produce vomiting, diarrhea, etc."

Spallanzani fertilized a frog's egg with 1-2,984,687,500 part of a grain of the seminal fluid of frogs.

It has been estimated that a cubic inch would contain 125 sextillions of bacteria or, in other words, 125 followed by twenty-one cyphers. Yet each one is a living thing.

Let us take another view: Analyses show that three and a half ounces of blood cells contain normally the mineral constituents in these proportions, viz.: Iron phos., 0.998; potass. sulph., 0.132; potass. chloride, 3.079; potass. phos., 2.343; sodium phos., 0.633; sodium chloride, 0.344; calcium phos., 0.094; mag. phos, 0.060, which stated relatively to each other in percentages is, iron phos., 12.98; potass sulph., 1.71; potass. chloride, 40.07; potass. phos., 30.50; sod. phos. 8.23; sod. chlor., 4.47; cal. phos., 1.22; mag. phos., .78.

The ascertained waste of all the Cell-Salts is about one ounce every 24 hours. The average is 8-10 of an ounce, or 384 grains, which is 16 grains per hour, or a total of 256,000,000,000,000 atoms each hour.

These, distributed according to the proportions existing in the system would give as the normal loss per hour:

Ferr. phos........... 33,280,000,000,000 Atoms.
Pot. sulph.,............4,352,000,000,000
Pot. chor............102,400,000,000,000
Pot. phos............ 78,080,000,000,000
Sod. phos............ 21,120,000,000,000
Sod. chlor........... 11,520,000,000,000
Cal. phos............ 3,072,000,000,000
Mag. phos 2,048,000,000,000

Nearly all diseases are local in their origin, i. e., when from lack of iron congestion begins, not over one thousandth part of the body is involved at first.

The thousandth part of the iron molecules in the body equal 33,280,000,000, the deficiency of which, if estimated at 10 per cent. below the difference between working and subsistence diet (which is 48 per cent.) would be 1,597,440,000 molecules, which would be replaced by 2-10 of one dose of Ferr. Phos.

The above showing of the relative wastes of the Salts, very strongly suggests the propriety of dosing them relatively somewhat in proportion to their probable loss, but more investigation is needed in this direction.

But the objector says : " Certainly the higher potencies, the two hundredth for example, can contain no drug, it must be trituated all away." Answer : Doubtless, this is true of organic substances, but cannot be of the indestructible inorganic Salts, for what fire cannot burn away, the mortar cannot triturate away.

True, Dr. D., in the *Homeopathic News*, says, that "it disappears in the eighteenth trituration." Whether this be true or not, abstractly considered, as a practical element, it is doubtful whether it exists beyond the tenth, although there is satisfactory evidence to show that *something* cures even in much higher potencies.

There are supposed to be more than 1,200 million cells in the brain and spinal cord alone, each cell built up by these wonderful processes of Cell-Salt action.

The life of a blood corpuscle is supposed to be about six weeks. What that of other tissue cells is we know not, but these amazing changes going on continuously without a break through life show to the reflective mind the boundlessness of the wisdom that planned the structure, and the ceaseless watchfulness and power of the Providence that secures its perpetuity.

CHAPTER IV.

THE INDICATIONS OR SYMPTOMS THAT CALL FOR THE USE OF EACH CELL-SALT.

Under many symptoms two or more remedies are named. When this is the case, the one should be employed whose physiological properties as given in chapter III best agree with the particular help that nature needs, e. g., boils, Ferr. Phos., Kali. Mur., Calc. Sulph., Silica.

When heat and pain indicate congestion, Ferr. Phos.

When swelling sets in, Kali. Mur.

To prevent suppuration, Calc. Sulph.

This proving unavailing, to *hasten* suppuration, Silica.

Hence the practical rule should be : When two or more Salts are named for one symptom, give the one most strongly indicated, and if that fails, the next, and so on successively, or in alternation.

The following Combination Table is taken from Dr. Walker's work, and was prepared by Professor Carnelly, an eminent doctor of science, and is believed to be very accurate. For the sake of brevity numbers are attached instead of the names of the Salts :

No. 1. *Calcium Phosphate* may be combined (taken with) with Nos. 2, 3, 4, 5, 6, 8, 9, 10 and 12.

No. 2. *Calcium Sulphate* with Nos. 1, 3, 5, 7, 9, 11 and 12.

No. 3. *Calcium Fluoride* with Nos. 1, 2, 5, 9 and 12.

No. 4 *Ferric Phosphate* with Nos. 1, 5, 6, 7, 8, 9, 10, 11 and 12.

No. 5. *Potassium Chloride* with Nos. 1, 3, 4, 6, 7, 8, 9 and 12.

No. 6. *Potassium Phosphate* with Nos. 1, 4, 5, 7, 8, 10 and 12.

No. 7. *Potassium Sulphate* with Nos. 2, 5, 6, 8, 11 and 12.

No. 8. *Magnesium Phosphate* with Nos. 1, 4, 6,7, 9, 10, 11 and 12.

No. 9. *Sodium Chloride* with Nos. 1, 3, 5, 8, 10, 11 and 12

No. 10. *Sodium Phosphate* with Nos. 1, 4, 6, 8, 9, 11 and 12.

No. 11. *Sodium Sulphate* with Nos. 2, 7, 8, 9, 10 and 12.

No. 12. *Silica* with all.

It will be noticed that the *phosphates* combine with each other ; so, also, do the *sulphates*, and the *chlorides* and *fluorides*, while *silica* combines with all.

Do NOT FORGET that the special locality of the trouble is of no account in selecting a remedy only as it affords an opportunity for a symptom to be revealed, i. e., congestion whether in eye, throat, stomach, bowels, kidney, bladder or foot, calls for Ferr. Phos. ; and so of all the Salts—they are all constitutional, not local merely.

DOSAGE.—While making the suggestion on a previous page of the advisability of dosing the Salts somewhat according to their relative waste within a specified time, it is deemed best to adhere in this book to the customary three grain dosage, to be administered one to four times a day in chronic cases, and from once in ten minutes to once in two hours in acute cases, being governed by the violence of the symptoms.

Mag. Phos. should usually be given in hot water in acute cases.

All the other Salts should be also when a *very speedy* effect is desired.

When more convenient, the tablets or powder may be dissolved in water and given in spoonful doses, being careful to dissolve three grains for every teaspoonful prepared.

Tablets of this size   ⬤   are one grain.

Tablets of this size   ⬤   are three grains.

The Salts may be advantageously employed externally whenever so prescribed by dissolving one dose of the Salt to every teaspoonful of water used for the lotion.

Apply with a compress, and cover to prevent too rapid evaporation.

The powder, or tablets pulverized, may also be made into an *ointment* with olive oil or vaseline and used in appropriate cases.

No classification can be made that will not contain the same symptom, under different divisions, and thus duplicate the symptoms, e. g., neuralgia in the head, would naturally be found under *head, nerves and pain*, but in this book, the first principle of classification being the functions and the second the organs, it will fall under *Pain*, and if not found there, under the organs, i. e., *Nerves*, instead of in all three places, and thus save expense.

Section i—Circulation.

The function of circulation is :

1. To carry the blood with uniform regularity, volume and force to all the tissues. (See Arteries and Heart.)

2. To convey the wastes of the system to the excretory organs for expulsion. (See Veins and Excretion.)

ARTERIES—BLOOD—HEART—VEINS.

ARTERIES.

Aneurism (rupture of) in early stage, if Iodide of Potash has not been used, Calc. Fluor. and Ferrum Phos.

Calcareous deposits (Atheroma), Calc. Phos.

Hardening (Scleroma), Calc. Fluor. and Kali. Mur.

Inflammation of, acute (Arteritis), Ferrum Phos. and Kali. Phos.

Thickening of the walls (Arteritis Obliterans) Kali. Mur.

Throbbing of temporal artery; excited by least touch, Kali. Mur.

BLOOD.

Accumulated in blood vessels of any part, Ferrum Phos.

All diseases arising from disturbed circulation or abnormal condition of red blood corpuscles, Ferrum Phos.

Anæmia (bloodlessness), Calc. Phos. chief remedy; Nat. Mur. and Kali. Phos., according to characteristic symptoms.

Anæmia, caused by long-continued depression of the mind, Kali.Phos.

Anæmia, when improvement in general health is noted, Ferrum Phos.

Bleeding, blood bright red and easily coagulates, Ferrum Phos.

Bleeding, blood dark, black, clotted or tough, Kali. Mur.

Bleeding, dark, blackish, thin, not coagulating, Kali. Phos. and Nat. Mur.

Bleeding of gums, predisposition to, Kali. Phos.

Bleeding of wounds, Ferrum Phos. internally and externally, surgical aid if severe.

Bleeding, pale red, thin, watery, Nat. Mur.

Blood corpuscles, increase of white with decrease of red (Leukæmia), Ferrum Phos.

Blood vessels, inflammation of, Ferrum Phos.

Circulation easily agitated, Silica.

Circulation excited by every motion, Nat. Mur.

Circulation poor, Kali. Phos., Calc. Phos.

Circulation sluggish in nervous, sensitive persons, Kali. Phos.

Clotted blood blown from nose, Nat. Mur.

Congestion (Hyperæmia), Ferrum Phos.

Dilatation of blood-vessels, Calc. Fluor., Ferrum Phos.

Excessive quantity of (Plethora), Nat. Sulph. and abstinence ; sweat baths in bad cases.

Hands and feet cold, Nat. Mur., Calc. Phos.

Hemorrhage from bladder or urethra, Ferrum Phos.

Hemorrhage from nose, stomach, bowels or lungs, Ferrum Phos.

Hemorrhage from nose at night, Kali. Mur.

Hemorrhage from nose before menses, Nat. Sulph.

Hemorrhage from nose in delicate persons, Kali. Phos.

Hemorrhage from nose in afternoon, Calc. Phos.

Hemorrhage from nose in place of chill, Nat. Mur.

Hemorrhage from nose in children, Ferrum Phos.

Hemorrhage from nose, predisposition to, in debilitated cases, Nat. Mur , Kali. Phos., Ferrum Phos.

Hemorrhage from nose, predisposition to, in appoplectic persons, Ferrum Phos.

Hemorrhage from nose, relieves headache, Ferrum Phos.

Hemorrhage from nose, when stooping or coughing, Nat. Mur.

Poison, Ferrum Phos. and Kali. Sulph. frequently, and in large doses.   Colon flush.

Poverty of (Anæmia), Calc. Phos., Ferrum Phos.

Poverty of, from depressing influences ; nervousness, Kali. Phos.

Pulse intermittent, irregular, from exhausting causes ; Kali. Phos.

Rushes to head, Ferrum Phos.

Tendency to form fibrinous clots (Embolus), Kali. Mur.

Throbbing in blood vessels, Silica.

Vomiting of dark, clotted blood, Kali. Mur.

HEART.

Beating of irregular, Nat. Mur.

Beating of irregular, worse lying on left side, Nat. Mur.

Beating of perceptible, but not hastened, Kali. Mur.

Beating of felt in nape of neck and left chest while sitting, Calc. Phos.

Beats slow and full, then quick and weak, Nat. Mur.

Beats quickened by slightest motion, Nat. Mur.

Chronic valvular disease of, Nat. Mur.

Cold feeling about when exerting the mind, Nat. Mur.

Cold feeling in region of, Kali Mur.

Congestion of, Ferrum Phos.

Constriction of, intermittent pulse, lower lungs oppressed, Nat. Mur.

Cutting, shooting in region of, interrupts breathing, Calc. Phos.

Dilation of, or of blood vessels, Calc. Fluor.

Disease of, causing dropsy, Calc. Phos., Ferrum Phos., Nat. Mur.

Enlargement of, Kali. Mur.

Enlargement of, caused by increased nutritive activity, Nat. Mur., Calc. Fluor.

Excessive action of (aneurism), Ferrum Phos.
Fainting from any cause, Kali. Phos.
Fluttering of, worse lying down, Nat. Mur.
Fluttering of, with weak, faint feeling, Nat. Mur.
Heart-burn after meals, Calc. Phos.
Inflammation of, Ferrum Phos.
Inflammation of, second stage, Kali. Mur.
Intense pain in (angina pectoris), Mag. Phos.
Intermittent action of, Kali. Phos.
Overworked, Nat. Mur.
Pain from front of down to thigh, Calc. Sulph.
Palpitation after rheumatic fever, Kali. Phos.
Palpitation and heat on waking, Silica.
Palpitation during exertion, Nat. Mur.
Palpitation from congestion, Ferrum Phos.
Palpitation from excessive flow of blood, Kali. Mur.
Palpitation from going up stairs, Kali. Phos., Nat. Phos.
Palpitation from indigestion, Nat. Phos.
Palpitation from nervous causes, Kali. Phos., Silica.
Palpitation from strange noise, Ferrum Phos.
Palpitation in debilitated persons, with watery blood, Nat. Mur.
Palpitation, spasmodic, Mag. Phos.
Palpitation, violent after quick motion, Silica.
Palpitation when lying on left side, Nat. Mur.
Palpitation when going to sleep or awaking, Nat. Mur.
Palpitation while sitting, compels holding on to something, Silica.
Palpitation while standing or ascending steps, Nat. Mur.
Palpitation with anxiety and sadness, Nat. Mur., Calc. Phos.
Palpitation with anxiety followed by weak trembling, Kali. Phos., Calc. Phos.

Palpitation with constriction of chest, Kali. Mur., Nat. Mur.

Palpitation with hysteria, Nat. Mur.

Palpitation with morning headache, Nat. Mur.

Palpitation with short breath, Kali. Phos.

Pressure about, Nat. Sulph.

Pulsations full, Ferrum Phos.

Pulsations felt in different parts of body, Nat. Phos.

Pulsations hard, small, rapid, Silica.

Pulsations imperceptible, Silica.

Pulsations intermittent, Kali. Phos, Nat. Mur.

Pulsations intermit every third beat, Nat. Mur.

Pulsations intermit every 25th or 30th beat, Kali. Mur.

Pulsations irregular, intermitting when lying on left side, Nat. Mur.

Pulsations increased, Ferrum Phos.

Pulsations irregular and slow, Silica.

Pulsations irregular and intermittent, Kali. Phos.

Pulsations quick and weak, or full and slow, Nat. Mur.

Pulsations rapid and intermittent, Nat. Mur.

Pulsations soft, sluggish, not corresponding with heart beats, Kali. Mur.

Pulsations shake whole body, Nat. Mur.

Severe pressure below heart after retiring, Nat. Mur.

Sharp pains in, interrupt breathing, Calc. Phos.

Sharp, shooting, darting pains, Mag. Phos.

Sinking spells in wasting fevers, Kali. Phos.

Stitches in after reading aloud, Nat. Mur.

Trembling about, worse ascending steps or after eating, Nat. Phos.

Troubles from nervous exhaustion, Silica.

Uneasiness about, Nat. Sulph.

Weak, Kali. Phos.

Weak from engorgement, Calc. Fluor.

VEINS.

Feel full as if would burst, Calc. Fluor.

Inflammation of, Ferrum Phos., Kali Sulph.

Varicose, Calc. Fluor., Ferrum Phos.

Varicose ulceration of, Calc. Fluor., also as a lotion on lint.

SECTION 2—ELIMINATION AND EXCRETION.

It is the function of elimination to separate from the tissue-cells all the worn out and useless matters, and of excretion to expel them from the system.

BOWELS—GLANDS—LIVER—MUCUS MEMBRANE—SKIN—
TISSUE CELLS—URINARY ORGANS.

BOWELS.

Anus, abscess about, with fistula, Calc. Sulph.

Anus, bearing down towards, Calc. Phos.

Anus, burning in after stool, Nat. Mur., Nat. Sulph, Silica.

Anus, burning, itching and stitches in, Silica.

Anus, constricted feeling in during stool, Silica.

Anus, constricting, lancinating in during stool, Nat. Mur.

Anus, crampy pains from, into rectum and testicles, Silica.

Anus, dryness and smarting in, Nat. Mur.

Anus, eruption about, Nat. Mur.

Anus, fistula with pains in joints in cold, damp weather, Calc. Phos.

Anus, fistula with chest symptoms, Silica.

Anus, fissures of, Calc. Phos. Calc. Fluor.

Anus, fissures of, in children, Calc. Phos.

Anus, itching of, worse in evening, Calc. Phos.
Anus, itching of, from worms, Nat. Phos.
Anus, pains during stool, as if constricted, Silica.
Anus, prolapse of, Calc. Fluor., Nat. Mur., Nat. Sulph. Silica.
Anus, pulsating warmth in, Calc. Phos.
Anus, smarting in with diarrhea, Nat. Sulph.
Anus, sore on rising in morning, Calc. Phos.
Anus, sore when walking, Nat. Mur.
Anus, sore, raw, itching, Nat. Phos.
Anus, syphilis in, Kali. Mur.
Anus, torn, contracted, bleeding, Nat. Mur.
Anus, wart-like eruptions on and between thighs, Nat. Sulph.
Burning in, Nat Mur.
Burning in, rising into chest and throat, Calc. Phos.
Bruised pain in, Nat. Sulph.
Cholera, Inflammatory state, Ferrum Phos.
Cholera, in drunkards, Nat. Mur.
Cholera in drunkards, second stage ; nerves of intestinal canal affected, Kali. Phos., Mag. Phos.
Chronic catarrh of, Nat. Mur.
Colic before stool, Ferrum Phos.
Colic better after stool, Nat. Sulph.
Colic bilious with belching and pain, Nat. Mur., Nat. Sulph.
Colic bilious with vomiting of bile, bitter taste, Nat. Sulph.
Colic during stool, Silica.
Colic daily attacks of, Mag. Phos.
Colic flatulent, better from bending double, Kali Phos., Mag. Phos.
Colic, flatulent, umbilical region, Mag. Phos.

Colic flatulent, or labor-like, Nat. Mur. Nat. Phos.

Colic flatulent, remittant, gripes, crampy pains, Mag. Phos.

Colic flatulent, relieved by friction, warmth and eructation, Mag. Phos.

Colic flatulent, of children and the new-born, Mag. Phos.

Colic from constipation, Silica.

Colic from sudden changes, Kali. Sulph.

Colic from worms, Nat. Phos., Silica.

Colic griping after stool, Nat. Phos.

Colic griping in intestines after eating, Kali. Phos.

Colic in children, with green or sour-smelling stools, Nat. Phos.

Colic menstrual, Mag. Phos.

Colic of infants, Mag. Phos.

Colic with diarrhea, Calc. Sulph.

Colic with nausea, better after passing wind, Nat. Mur.

Colic with pain in small of back as if bruised; better lying on side, Nat. Sulph.

Colic with reddish, bloody stools, Silica.

Colic with rumbling, Calc. Sulph.

Colic with yellow hands and blue nails, Silica.

Colicky pain in right groin, extending over whole abdomen, Nat. Sulph.

Constant rumbling in, Kali. Phos.

Constant urging to stool, Kali. Mur.

Constipation accompanied by drowsiness, Nat. Mur.

Constipation accompanied by dull, heavy headache, Nat. Mur.

Constipation alternating with diarrhea, Nat. Mur.

Constipation alternating with mushy stool, Nat. Mur., Nat. Sulph.

Constipation during consumption, Calc. Sulph.

Constipation from debility of muscular fibers, Ferr. Phos.

Constipation from dryness of mucus lining, with watery secretions elsewhere, Nat. Mur.

Constipation from inactivity of rectum, Nat. Mur., Kali. Phos.

Constipation from piles, Nat. Mur.

Constipation from sluggish liver, stools light colored, Kali. Mur.

Constipation habitual with coated tongue, Kali. Sulph.

Constipation in poorly nourished children, Silica.

Constipation of old people and infants, Calc. Phos.

Constipation with dizziness and dull headache, Calc. Phos.

Constipation with hectic fever and difficult breathing, Calc. Sulph.

Constipation with heat in rectum or hard feces, Ferr. Phos.

Constipation with large slime covered feces, Silica.

Constipation with spinal affections as if rectum was paralyzed, Salica.

Constipation with piles or prolapsus of rectum, Ferr. Phos.; Calc. Fluor.

Constipation with light-colored stools, Kali. Mur.

Constipation with uterine displacements, Nat. Mur.

Constipation with white or grayish-white tongue, Kali. Mur.

Cramps and wind colic, often with watery diarrhea, Mag. Phos.

Cutting and griping with rumbling in abdomen, Nat. Mur.

Cutting pain in region of navel, through to back, Silica.

Depression of mind with hard stool, Calc. Phos.

Diarrhea after exposure to cold air, Silica.

Diarrhea after fatty food, pastry, etc., Kali. Mur.

Diarrhea after use of opium, Nat. Mur.

Diarrhea after vexation, Calc. Phos.

Diarrhea after vaccination, Silica.

Diarrhea causes soreness and smarting, Nat. Mur.

Diarrhea chronic, Calc. Phos., Ferr. Phos., Nat. Mur., Nat. Sulph., Silica.

Diarrhea from eating fruit, vegetables, pastry, cold food or drink, Nat. Sulph.

Diarrhea from excess of acidity, Nat. Phos.

Diarrhea from fright or depressing causes, Kali. Phos.

Diarrhea from juicy fruit or cider, Calc. Phos.

Diarrhea from ulceration of bowels, Silica.

Diarrhea in morning before rising, Silica.

Diarrhea in teething children, Calc. Phos.

Diarrhea offensive, carrion-like stools, Kali. Phos.

Diarrhea of children, Calc. Phos., Nat. Mur., Nat. Sulph., Silica.

Diarrhea of scrawny children, sweaty head and offensive foot sweat, Silica.

Diarrhea of school girls, Calc. Phos.

Diarrhea on rising, sudden urging, much wind, Nat. Sulph.

Diarrhea painful, passes nothing but mucus, Kali. Mur.

Diarrhea painless, watery, Kali. Phos., Nat. Mur.

Diarrhea slight, with painful urging before stool, Calc. Fluor.

Diarrhea very offensive, Calc. Phos., Kali. Phos.

Diarrhea watery, weakening, Silica.

Diarrhea while eating, sudden, imperative, Kali. Phos.

Diarrhea with emaciation, prostration and passing of undigested food, Ferr. Phos., Calc. Phos.

Diarrhea with flatulence, Calc. Phos.

Diarrhea with great thirst, Silica, Nat. Mur.

Diarrhea with heavy odor, Kali. Phos.

Diarrhea with pain in abdomen after eating maple sugar, or change in weather, Calc. Sulph.

Diarrhea with pinching pain from navel to back, Mag. Phos.

Diarrhea with painful urging before stool, Calc. Phos.

Diarrhea with red, itching, restless feet in evening, Mag. Phos.

Diarrhea with suppressed urine, Silica.

Diarrhea with vomiting, and cramps in calves, Kali. Phos., Mag. Phos.

Diarrhea worse after floury food, Nat. Mur.

Diarrhea worse after motion, Nat. Mur., Nat. Sulph.

Diarrhea worse in cold, damp weather, Nat. Sulph.

Diarrhea in morning after moving about, Nat. Mur.

Diarrhea watery, involuntary, painless stools, fever, thirst, Nat. Mur.

Dysentery, colon flush of hot water as local remedy.

Dysentery, bloody stools every fifteen minutes, cutting pain, severe straining, Kali. Mur.

Dysentery, sharp, griping pain, Mag. Phos.

Dysentery, violent fever, pain worse on pressure of stomach, Ferr. Phos.

Dysentery with pus-like slime, Calc. Sulph.

Dysentery with pus and much blood, Kali. Mur., Calc. Sulph.

Dysentery with cramping pain, better from bending double, friction or warmth, Mag. Phos.

Flatus (wind) fears to pass lest feces escape, Nat. Phos.

Flatus, passing of, Calc. Phos., Mag. Phos.

Flatus noisy, Kali. Phos.

Flatus offensive, Calc. Phos., Kali. Phos.

Flatus offensive, large quantities after meals, loose stools, Nat. Sulph.

Gnawing in, Mag. Phos.

Great torpor of without pain, Nat. Mur., Kali. Phos.

Griping in, relieved by kneading, Nat. Sulph.

Grumbling and rolling, followed by diarrhea, Nat. Sulph.

Heat in lower bowel, with green, bilous discharge, Nat. Sulph.

Neuralgia of, Mag. Phos.

Pain, dead, heavy from bowels to back, Nat Sulph.

Pain causes restless sleep, Nat. Phos.

Pains relieved by pressure, rubbing or warmth, Mag. Phos.

Piles, bleeding, Calc. Fluor.

Piles, bleeding, bright red blood, Ferr. Phos.

Piles, bleeding, dark, thick blood, Kali Mur.

Piles, cutting, darting, lightning-like pains, Mag. Phos.

Piles, for Pain and soreness, Calc. Fluor., Ferr. Phos.

Piles, itching, Calc. Phos., Calc. Fluor., Ferr. Phos.

Piles, protrusion of, Calc. Phos., Silica, Calc. Fluor.

Piles, sore, painful and itching, Kali. Phos. Ferr. Phos., Nat. Mur.

Piles, very painful, crampy pains from rectum to anus or testicles, Silica.

Piles, with bloody mucous from rectum, Silica.

Piles, catarrh of stomach and bowels, Ferr. Phos.

Piles, catarrh of stomach and yellow mucous-coated tongue, Kali. Sulph.

Piles, swelling, and burning pain, Kali. Phos.

Piles, stinging pain, oozing from rectum, eruptions about anus, Nat. Mur.

Pinching in, with, pain in forehead ; rumbling, shifting pain, followed by diarrhea, Nat. Sulph.

Pressure on bladder and rectum before stool, Nat. Mur.

Pulsating, burning and warmth in anus and rectum, Nat. Mur.

Rectum, burning pain in, Nat. Mur.

Rectum, burning and scratching in during stool, Silica, Nat. Mur.

Rectum, constant pains in, Kali, Mur.

Rectum, cutting, jerking, dull stinging pain, Silica.

Rectum, feels like foreign body in ; constant looseness, Nat. Mur.

Rectum, inactivity of causes constipation, Nat. Mur., Silica.

Rectum, sharp stitches in when walking, Silica.

Seat worms, Nat. Mur.

Smarting and dryness of anus and rectum, Nat. Mur.

Sore and tender, Ferr. Phos.

Stools, black, watery, Nat. Mur.

Stools, black, thin, offensive, Kali. Sulph.

Stools, bleeding with or after, followed by slime, Calc. Phos.

Stools, blood passes with slime in dysentery, Kali. Mur.

Stools, bloody or bloody mucous, Ferr. Phos., Kali. Mur.

Stools, buzzing in ears after, Calc. Phos.

Stools, chronic, soft, Nat. Mur.

Stools, chilliness and nausea in throat during, Silica.

Stools, clay-colored, Kali. Mur., Nat. Phos , Nat. Sulph.

Stools, wind, urging, straining after breakfast, Kali. Phos.

Stools, come to verge of anus and then slip back, Silica.

Stools, contain undigested food; great prostration, Silica, Ferr. Phos.

Stools, contraction in rectum and urethra before, Nat. Mur.

Stools, cutting abdominal pains before, Nat. Mur.

Stools, dark or green bile, Nat. Sulph.

Stools, desire for every few minutes, Calc. Phos., Kali. Mur.

Stools, desire for frequent, ineffectual, Nat. Mur.

Stools, difficult expulsions, leaving much soreness, Nat. Mur., Silica.

Stools, dry and hard, Nat. Mur.

Stools, expelled with force, Mag. Phos., Nat. Sulph.

Stools, first part natural, last part loose, Calc. Fluor., Nat. Phos.

Stools, frequent, green, watery; mixed with mucous; slimy, Ferr. Phos., Calc. Phos.

Stools, frequent, scanty, liquid, offensive, Silica, Kali. Phos.

Stools, frothy, black, watery, Nat. Mur.

Stools, greenish, thin, of children; sometimes slimy, Nat. Phos.

Stools, green or white with jaundice, Nat. Phos.

Stools, green, skin and eyes yellow, Nat. Sulph.

Stools, green, sour, Nat. Phos., Silica.

Stools, green, watery or hashed; scanty; mucous, Ferr. Phos.

Stools, gushing, Nat. Sulph.

Stools, hard, dry, crumbling, Nat. Mur.

Stools, hard, dark, after breakfast, Kali. Phos.

Stools, hard, lumpy, clay-like, expelled with great difficulty, Nat. Sulph., Silica.

Stools, hard in old people, causing vertigo, Calc. Phos.

Stools, hard, with mental depression, Calc. Phos.

Stools, hot and watery, Calc. Phos.

Stools, hot and offensive, Calc. Phos., Kali. Phos.

Stools, in large masses, Nat. Mur.

Stools, involuntary; when passing wind, Nat. Mur., Nat. Sulph.

Stools, irregular, hard, unsatisfactory, Nat. Mur.

Stools, labor-like pains during; better by pressure, Nat. Mur.

Stools, large, soft, with loss of expulsive power, Silica, Calc. Fluor.

Stools, like bloody fish-brine, Nat. Phos.

Stools, like rice water, Kali. Phos.

Stools, like sheep's dung, Nat. Mur.

Stools, light-colored from want of bile, Kali. Mur.

Stools, loose, watery, urging, Mag. Phos., Nat. Sulph.

Stools, mucous, followed by itching of anus; mushy, offensive, Silica, Kali. Phos.

Stools natural, but difficult and painful, Silica.

Stools, obstinate retention of, Nat. Mur.

Stools, offensive, undigested, dark, loose, followed by uneasy urging, Kali. Phos., Ferr. Phos.

Stools, only in five to seven days, then after artificial means, Silica.

Stools, pains after, Calc. Phos.

Stools, pains in bowels before, Ferr. Phos., Nat. Mur., Nat. Sulph., Silica.

Stools, pale yellow, clay colored, Kali. Mur.

Stools, pure blood, bloody mucus or pus, Ferr. Phos., Kali. Phos.

Stools, remain a long time in anus, Silica.

Stools, soft, passed with difficulty, Calc. Phos., Nat. Sulph., Silica.

Stools, straining and retching during, moans, rolls head, face pinched, urine scanty, Ferr. Phos.

Stools, torn feeling after, Nat. Mur.

Stools, transparent, glassy, like white of egg, Nat. Mur.

Stools, undigested in children with skull bones not grown up, Silica.

Stools, watery, weakening, Silica, Nat. Mur.

Stools, watery, with much wind, Nat. Sulph.

Stools, white and mushy, Calc. Phos.

Stools, white, watery, like whey; tongue dry; no thirst; cramps, Nat. Mur.

Stools, with pinching in groins and stomach before, Nat. Sulph.

Stools, yellowish green, Nat. Sulph.

Summer complaint, Calc. Phos.

Sulphurous odor of gas from, Kali. Sulph.

Symptoms cease when mind is employed, Kali. Phos.

Tendency to prolapsed rectum, Calc. Phos., Calc. Fluor.

Ulceration of, Nat. Phos., Calc. Sulph.

Uneasiness in and constant urging to stool, Nat. Phos., Nat. Sulph.

GLANDS.

Of armpit, swollen and sore, Kali. Mur.

Of armpit, swollen and suppurating, Calc. Sulph., Silica.

Enlarged, chronic, Kali. Mur. and Calc. Phos., intercurrently.

Glandular swellings, Kali. Mur., chief remedy; if very hard, Calc. Fluor.

Glands and gums swollen, Kali. Mur.
Glands, swelling of, under tongue, Nat. Mur.
Lymphatic, suppuration threatening, Calc. Sulph.
Mumps, for first stage, and pain, Ferr. Phos.
Mumps, for swelling, Kali. Mur., alternated with Ferr. Phos.
Mumps, with excessive secretion of saliva, or swelling of testicles, Nat. Mur., intercurrently.
Mumps, without fever, Kali. Mur.
Of neck, enlarged, sore when coughing, Nat. Mur.
Of neck, painful, sore, Calc. Phos.
Of neck, stony, hard, Calc. Fluor.
Of neck, swollen, Kali. Mur., Silica.
Of neck, swollen, chronic, Nat. Sulph.
Of neck, swelling of, extends to chest, Nat. Phos.
Salivary glands enlarged and tender, Kali. Mur.

LIVER.

Liver affections with nerve depression, Kali. Phos.
Liver, beating-soreness in, worse in motion or lying on right side, Silica.
- Liver, biliousness from mental overwork, Nat Sulph. and Kali. Phos.
Liver, biliousness from too much bile, Nat. Sulph.
Liver, enlargement of, Nat. Sulph.
Liver, enlargement of, pain in right side, emptiness of stomach ; white or gray tongue, Kali. Mur.
Liver, gall-stones, to prevent reformation, Calc. Phos., Nat. Sulph.
Liver, induration of, Silica.
Liver, irritable, after mental work, Nat. Sulph., Kali. Phos.
Liver, jaundice after vexation, Nat. Sulph.

Liver, jaundice from a chill, catarrh of duodenum, Kali. Mur.

Liver, jaundice from stomach catarrh, drowsiness and watery secretions, Nat. Mur.

Liver, jaundice with greenish brown tongue, sallow skin or yellow eye-balls, Nat. Sulph.

Liver, jaundice with malarial symptoms, Nat. Sulph.

Liver, jaundice with drowsiness, Nat. Mur.

Liver, left lobe enlarged, Mag. Phos.

Liver, sensitive, Nat. Sulph.

Liver, sluggish, with white or gray tongue and light-colored stools, Kali. Mur.

Liver, swollen and sore to touch, Nat. Sulph.

Liver, swollen, skin earthy, sallow, infiltrated, Nat. Mur.

Liver, thickening of, especially with succession of boils, Nat. Phos.

Liver troubles, with chronic constipation, Silica.

Liver, torpor of, Kali. Mur.

MUCOUS MEMBRANES.

Acrid, corroding discharge, Silica.

Bland, watery coryza, worse in morning, Kali. Phos.

Blisters on palate, Nat. Sulph.

Blisters on tip of tongue, Nat. Mur., Calc. Phos.

Blistered mouth and lips, Kali. Sulph.

Blood-blisters on inside of lips, bloody saliva, Nat. Mur.

Blood-streaked mucous in nose after a bath, Calc. Sulph.

Burning and dryness of mouth, nose, etc., Nat. Sulph.,

Burning in nose, internal soreness, pimples inside, Nat. Mur.

Catarrh accompanied by fever, Ferr. Phos.

Catarrh, acute or chronic, with slimy, yellow, greenish discharge, Kali. Sulph.

Catarrh, acute, first stage, Ferr. Phos.

Catarrh, acute, fluent, alternating with stoppage, Nat. Mur.

Catarrh, acute, fluent in cold room, stopped out of doors and in warm air, Calc. Phos.

Catarrh, acute, fluent with sneezing, Nat. Mur., Silica.

Catarrh, acute stage of resolution, Calc. Sulph.

Catarrh, acute, thick, yellow, lumpy, mattery discharge, Kali. Sulph., Calc. Sulph.

Catarrh, acute, unbearable in open air, Silica.

Catarrh, acute, watery, excoriating discharge, worse in open air, Calc. Sulph.

Catarrh, acute, with albuminous (white of egg) discharge, Calc. Phos.

Catarrh, acute, with dry harsh skin, Kali. Sulph.

Catarrh, acute, with mattery, slimy discharge, Nat. Mur.

Catarrh, aggravated in evening or warm room, Kali. Sulph.

Catarrh, bronchial, with difficult expectoration of tiny yellow lumps of mucus, Calc. Fluor.

Catarrh, cannot uncover head without taking cold, Silica.

Catarrh, chronic in scrofulous children, Calc. Phos.

Catarrh, chronic, smelling as of blood, Silica.

Catarrh, chronic, with pus discharge, Kali. Sulph., Silica.

Catarrh, chronic, with yellowish, viscous secretion, Kali. Sulph.

Catarrh, dry or stuffy, cough dry, tickling, or with yellow and bloody sputa ; voice hoarse, breathing oppressed, Kali. Mur.

Catarrh, nasal, after washing in cold water, Calc. Sulph.

Catarrh, nasal, better in open air, Calc. Phos., Kali. Sulph.

Catarrh, nasal, bones diseased, with offensive odor, Calc. Fluor.

Catarrh, nasal, congestion of nasal membranes, Ferr. Phos.

Catarrh, nasal, discharges when in a cold room or open air, Calc. Phos.

Catarrh, nasal, nose stopped on rainy days, Calc. Phos.

Catarrh, nasal, sensitive to air, Silica.

Catarrh of bladder, acute or chronic, Kali. Mur.

Catarrh of bladder, when secreting watery, transparent fluid, Nat. Mur.

Catarrh of bladder, with vomiting, pale face, loss of strength, dry tongue, Kali. Phos.

Catarrh of bronchi (acute), Silica.

Catarrh of bronchi in debilitated persons (chronic), Nat. Mur.

Catarrh of bronchi in scrofulous or gouty constitutions, Calc. Phos.

Catarrh of debilitated persons, Nat. Mur., Calc. Phos.

Catarrh of ear, involving eustachian tubes, Kali. Sulph.

Catarrh of middle ear, Ferr. Phos., Kali. Mur

Catarrh of ear with discharge of thin, yellow, greenish matter, Kali. Sulph. ; also daily injections of same in tepid water.

Catarrhal affections of ear, often combined with catarrh of the chest or bowels, Ferr. Phos.

Catarrhal inflammation (chronic), acrid discharge, Nat. Mur.

Catarrhal inflammation frontal cavities, Kali. Mur.

Catarrhal inflammation, mouth and pharynx, with watery discharge, Nat. Mur.

Catarrhal inflammation, stomach, causing jaundice, Kali. Sulph.

Catarrhal inflammation, stomach, chronic, yellow, slimy coated tongue, Kali. Sulph.

Catarrh, offensive smelling, Silica, Calc. Fluor.

Catarrh, stopped nose at night from head uncovered during the day, Nat. Mur.

Catarrh, takes cold easily, Ferr. Phos.

Catarrh with acid symptoms, Nat. Phos.

Catarrh with alternate dry and moist coryza, Mag. Phos.

Catarrh with brown, liquid, mustard looking dry tongue, Kali. Phos.

Catarrh with creamy, golden-yellow, moist coating, Nat. Phos.

Catarrh with dirty, brownish or grayish, green, slimy coat, Nat. Sulph.

Catarrh with excessive chronic dryness, or ulceration of edges of nostrils, Silica.

Catarrh with fever, Ferr. Phos.

Catarrh with gushing flow from nostrils, Mag. Phos.

Catarrh with influenza and sneezing, Nat. Mur.

Catarrh with itching of tip of nose, Silica.

Catarrh with Lagrippe, Nat. Sulph.

Catarrh with loss or perversion of smell, Mag. Phos.

Catarrh with loss of smell and taste, Nat. Mur.

Catarrh with offensive discharge, Kali. Phos.

Catarrh with offensive smell when not located in the bone, Silica.

Catarrh with red tongue, Ferr. Phos.

Catarrh with salty mucus, Nat. Mur.

Catarrh with stuffy sensation, dry, Kali. Mur.

Catarrh with white, not transparent, phlegm, Kali. Mur.

Catarrh with watery discharge, Nat. Mur.

Catarrh with whitish or gray-coated tongue, Kali. Mur.

Catarrh with yellow, slimy, sometimes whitish edge, Kali. Sulph.

Catarrh, worse at seaside, Nat. Mur., Nat. Sulph.

Catarrh, worse in changeable weather and when snow melts, Calc. Phos.

Cold in head, Nat. Mur. and Ferrum Phos.

Cold in head, fever blisters, Nat. Mur.

Cold in head, with collection of greenish mucous, Kali. Sulph., Silica.

Cold in head, with yellow, lumpy, green discharges, Calc. Fluor.

Constant spitting of frothy mucous, Nat. Mur.

Crusts in nose, Silica.

Crusts yellow, blown from nose, Kali. Phos.

Discharge, albuminous, Calc. Phos.

Discharge, bloody or white frothy mucous, in clots in morning, sourish, Nat. Mur.

Discharge, bloody and watery, Calc. Sulph.

Discharge, cheesy lumps coughed up, Kali. Mur.

Discharge, clear blood in pneumonia, Ferr. Phos.

Discharge, clear, tough white phlegm from back of palate, Nat. Phos.

Discharge, clear, mattery, transparent, Nat. Mur.

Discharge, foul from nose from affections of bone coverings or sub-mucous connective tissue, Silica.

Discharge, foul from nose from syphilitic affections, Nat. Sulph.

Discharge, from eyes of mucous or muco-pus, Nat. Mur.

Discharge, from eyes of mucous with suppuration, Silica.

Discharge from ears after use of mercury, Silica.

Discharge from ears brown, offensive from right, Kali. Sulph.

Discharge from ears curdy, watery, without pain except after fresh cold, Silica.

Discharge from ears excoriating, Calc. Phos.

Discharge from ears foul, thin, serous, greenish, offensive, Kali. Phos.

Discharge from ears mattery, watery, Kali. Sulph.

Discharge from ears mixed with blood, Kali. Phos.

Discharge from ears, of bloody mucous, Silica.

Discharge from ears offensive, purulent, Silica.

Discharge from ears, of pus, Calc. Phos., Kali. Sulph., Nat. Mur., Silica.

Discharge from ears thick, white and moist, Kali. Mur.

Discharge from ears thick, yellow, bloody, Calc. Sulph.

Discharge from ears, of thin yellow fluid, Kali. Sulph.

Discharge from navel, yellowish, with peculiar odor, Nat. Mur.

Discharge of offensive matter from opening at the roots of teeth, Silica.

Discharge, golden, yellow, creamy, Nat. Phos.

Discharge, greasy tasting, Silica.

Discharge like uncooked white of egg, Calc. Phos.

Discharge, mattery expectoration, Calc. Sulph.

Discharge, mucus slips back and may be swallowed, Kali. Sulph.

Discharge, mucus in throat and rattling in chest, Ferr. Phos.

Discharge, offensive, with nervous symptoms, Kali. Phos.

Discharge of yellow mucus, wakens from sleep, must clear it away, Nat. Phos.

Discharge only during day, Silica.

Discharge, phlegm loose, rattling, raised with difficulty, Nat. Mur.

Discharge, salty mucus hawked up, Nat. Mur., Nat. Sulph.

Discharge sticky, milky, acrid, purulent, sinks in water, Silica.

Discharge thick white or yellowish white, slimy, Kali. Mur.

Discharge thick lumpy green, Calc. Fluor.

Discharge thick, yellow, greenish, serous, slimy, Kali. Sulph.

Discharge thick green, yellow mucus or yellow offensive balls, Silica.

Discharge thick, milk-white, tenacious phlegm, white tongue, Kali. Mur.

Discharge thick, lumpy, light yellow, or pus-like, Calc. Sulph.

Discharge thick, ropy, yellowish green, Nat. Sulph.

Discharge thick, yellow phlegm drops in night, Calc. Phos.

Discharge thick, yellow, salty, offensive, Kali. Phos.

Discharge tough, clear white phlegm drops with much hawking, Nat. Phos.

Discharge, transparent mucus in throat in morning, Nat. Mur.

Discharge tiny yellow, tough lumps of bad-smelling mucus, Calc. Fluor.

Discharge watery from any part, with lack of activity. in some other, Nat. Mur.

Discharge yellow, creamy or acid, Nat. Phos.

Discharge yellow, or blood-streaked mucous, pain in forehead, Silica.

Discharge yellow, mucous raised easily, Kali. Sulph.

Discharge yellowish-green mucous from lungs Kali. Sulph., Silica.

Discharge yellowish, thick in consumption, Kali. Phos., Silica.

Discharge yellow, thin or watery, profuse, Kali. Sulph.

Discharge yellow, watery, mixed with blood, Calc. Sulph.

Discharge yellowish-green, thick, profuse expectoration of sweetish, greasy taste in consumption, Silica.

Dropping of watery, salty mucous into throat, Nat. Mur., Calc. Phos.

Dropping of tough albuminous mucous, Calc. Phos.

Dryness of in any part, Nat. Mur.

Dryness of in nose with scabbing, Silica.

Exudation of white or gray substance on tonsils, etc., Kali. Mur.

Greenish looking scab blown from nose in morning, Nat. Sulph.

Hardened mucous causes stoppage of nose, sore when removed, Silica, Kali. Phos.

Hawking and spitting constant, Calc. Phos.

Hawking of salty mucous in the morning, Nat. Sulph.

Hawking up phlegm late in evening, at night and morning, with gagging, Calc. Phos., Nat. Sulph.

Irritation of membrane, red, hot, dry, Ferr. Phos.

Irritated condition of, Silica.

Irritation of in nose, Nat. Sulph.

Loose yellow rattling phlegm raised with difficulty, Kali. Sulph.

Membrane glazed, but not granulated, Nat. Mur.

Mouth, accumulation of mucous in, Silica.
Mouth and tongue dry, thirst in afternoon, Calc. Phos.
Mucous membrane swollen, Nat. Mur., Silica.
Much mucous from nose, ineffectual desire to sneeze, Calc. Fluor.
Mucous in throat at night, Nat. Sulph.
Nostrils, edges of inflamed, Silica.
Nostrils sore, Nat. Sulph.
Nostrils sore, scabs form after picking, Nat. Phos.
Patches on pharynx and fauces, Kali. Mur.
Pus from nose changes to green when exposed to light, Nat. Sulph.
Scabs in nose, Nat. Mur., Silica.
Soft palate, yellow, creamy, Nat. Phos.
Sore spot inside of cheek, Calc. Phos.
Tears flow when coughing, Nat. Mur.
Tear-duct, closed, Nat. Mur.
Tear-duct, fistula of, Silica.
Throat dry at night, Calc. Phos.
Thrush in children, Kali. Mur.
Thrush in children with much saliva, Nat. Mur.
Tongue, blisters on, Calc. Phos., Nat. Mur., Nat. Sulph.
Tongue, blisters, burning, stinging, Nat. Sulph.
Tonsils covered with transparent mucous, Nat. Mur.
Tonsils, yellow mucous, raw feeling, Nat. Phos.
Vesicles and ulcers in mouth and on tongue, Nat. Mur.
Windpipe dry, also larynx, Nat. Mur.

SKIN.

Acne, itches and burns only during the day, Silica.
Acne, in the young or debilitated, Calc. Phos.
Acne rosacea, Calc. Phos.
Barber's itch, Kali. Mur.
Beard, falling of, Nat. Mur.

Blebs, with bloody, watery contents, Kali. Phos.

Blisters from burns, Kali. Mur., use locally also.

Blisters, filled with lymph, Kali. Mur.

Blisters here and there, Nat. Sulph.

Blisters like pearls around mouth, Nat. Mur.

Blisters on margins of lips, Silica.

Blisters with clear, watery contents, Nat. Mur.

Blotches on face, come and go, Nat. Phos.

Bluish face, Nat. Phos.

Brownish, dirty-white complexion, Calc. Phos.

Brownish, crusts on, Silica.

Brown spots on hands, Nat. Mur.

Burns and scalds, first remedy, Ferr. Phos., locally also.

Burns and scalds, suppurating, Calc. Sulph.

Chafing of skin, Kali. Mur., Kali. Sulph., Nat. Phos.

Chafing of, in children, with bilious symptoms, Nat. Sulph.

Chafing of, with excoriations, especially if inclined to scab, tongue whitish, Kali. Mur.

Chafing or rawness of, in children, Kali. Mur.

Chapped hands or lips from cold, Kali. Mur.

Chapped lips, Calc. Fluor.

Cheeks red, face hot, Nat. Mur.

Chicken pox, for fever, Ferr. Phos.

Chicken pox, second stage, with white or greyish-white tongue, Kali. Mur..

Chicken pox, with watery symptoms, drowsiness, stupor, etc., Nat. Mur.

Chilbrains for the tingling, itching pain, Kali. Phos., Kali. Mur.

Chilblains recently contracted, Kali. Mur.

Chilblains when suppurating, Calc. Sulph. after Kali. Mur. If this does not heal, Silica.

Cold sweat on face, body cold, Calc. Phos.

Cold and clammy on face, Calc. Phos.

Cold sores, Calc. Fluor, Nat. Mur.

Copious scaling of scalp, Kali. Sulph.

Coppery face, covered with pimples, Calc. Phos.

Corns, Nat. Mur.

Cracking of skin, Silica.

Cracked lips, Nat. Mur.

Cracks between toes, violent itching, Nat. Mur.

Crusta lactea (scald head), Calc. Sulph., Nat. Phos.

Crusts on scalp, in edge of hair like peach gum, Nat. Mur.

Dandruff, white scales, Nat. Mur.

Dandruff, yellow scales, Kali. Sulph.

Dark brown or yellowish skin, Calc. Phos.

Delicate, pale, growing children, Calc. Phos.

Dirty-looking, dry, withered, chlorosis, Nat. Mur.

Disease of skin, with acidity, Nat. Phos.

Discharge from, albuminous (white of egg), Calc. Phos.

Discharge from, blood and pus, Calc. Sulph.

Discharge from, fetid, Kali. Phos.

Discharge from, thick, yellow pus, Silica.

Dry and cracked on hands, Nat. Mur.

Dry skin, moist on hands, Calc. Phos.

Dry and hot in fevers, Kali. Sulph.

Dryness of, with scaling, Kali. Sulph.

Eczema, Calc. Fluor in alternation with Kali. Mur.

Eczema after vaccination with bad vaccine, Kali. Mur.

Eczema, eruption of suddenly suppressed, Kali. Sulph.

Eczema from eating too much salt, Nat. Mur.

Eczema, moist and oozing, secretion more watery than viscid, Nat. Sulph.

Eczema of scalp, hands and forearm, Silica.

Eczema of scalp, exuding corroding fluid destroying the hair, Nat. Mur.

Eczema, raw and inflamed, Nat. Mur.

Eczema, scurfy, discharging corrosive fluid, Nat. Mur.

Eczema, vesicular, thick, white secretions, Kali. Mur.

Eczema with debility, dry, crusty affections, Calc. Phos.

Eczema with deranged uterine functions, Kali. Mur.

Eczema with nervous irritation, oversensitiveness, Kali. Phos.

Eczema with symptoms of acidity, yellow, honey-colored secretions, Nat. Phos.

Eczema with white scales, Nat. Mur.; also apply locally.

Eczema with yellow crusts, Calc. Phos.

Eczema, worse on edges of hair, genitals and legs, Nat. Mur.

Eczema with yellow or greenish discharges, Kali. Sulph.

Eruptions and ulcers on chin, Nat. Mur., Silica.

Eruptions about anus, Nat. Mur.

Eruptions, burning, itching, with pus-like moisture, Kali. Sulph.

Eruptions, bends of elbows and knees, Nat. Mur.

Eruptions, herpetic, Nat. Mur.

Eruptions, itchy, on children, Kali. Sulph.

Eruptions, itching, Nat. Mur.

Eruptions, itching in eyebrows, Nat. Mur.

Eruptions in armpit, Kali. Sulph.

Eruptions on forehead, pustules, Nat. Mur.

Eruptions on head, gluey discharge, matting the hair Nat. Mur.

Eruptions on scalp with thin scales, Silica.

Eruptions of blisters. Kali. Mur.

Eruptions, pustules, pimples discharging a white, watery substance, Kali. Mur.

Eruptions, scaly, better from warm water, Kali. Sulph.

Eruptions suddenly suppressed or receding, Kali. Sulph.

Eruptions, wart-like, Nat. Sulph.

Eruptions, with white-coated tongue and deranged menstrual period, Kali. Mur.

Eruptions, with white scales, Calc. Phos., Kali. Mur.

Erysipelas, for inflammation and pain, Ferrum Phos., Nat. Sulph.

Erysipelas, smooth, red, shiny, tingling or painful swelling, intense itching, Nat. Phos., Nat. Sulph.

Erysipelas, vesicular, or shingles, Kali. Mur.

Erysipelas, with intense fever and inflammatory symptoms, Ferrum Phos.

Erysipelas, with suppuration, deep-seated, Silica.

Expression of pain or suffering, sickly, Kali. Mur.

Face earthy, yellow color, Nat. Mur.

Face feels cold or numb, Calc. Phos.

Face flushed, cold sensation at nape of neck, Ferr. Phos.

Face pale, yellowish, Silica.

Face pale, sickly, sallow, Kali. Phos., Calc. Phos.

Face pale and pallid, Ferrum Phos.

Face pale, in diphtheria, Nat. Mur.

Face yellowish with leucorrhea, Nat. Mur.

Festers, gathering easily, Calc. Sulph., Silica.

Fistula, long-standing, Nat. Sulph.

Fistula, with blue border, Nat. Sulph.

Fissures of anus, Calc. Fluor.

Freckles, Calc. Phos.

Greasy, offensive smelling scales or crusts, Kali. Mur., Kali. Phos.
Greyish skin, lead-colored, Calc. Sulph.
Hair, brushing or combing causes sneezing, Silica.
Hair, falls when combed, Calc. Sulph.
Hair, falling of, scalp sensitive, face shiny, oily, Nat. Mur.
Hair, poor crop of, Calc. Phos.
Hair, premature falling, Silica.
Hands, cracks in palms of, Calc. Fluor.
Head, bald spots on, Calc. Phos.
Herpes about the mouth, limbs and thighs, Nat. Mur.
Herpes in bends of elbows and knees, Nat. Mur,
Herpes, humid, on scrotum and thighs, Nat. Mur.
Herpes, moist, oozing, Nat. Mur.
Hives on face and body before ulceration of jaw, Silica.
Hives, itching all over like insect bites, Nat. Phos.
Hives, with harsh, dry skin, Calc. Fluor.
Hives, white, itching, red after rubbing, Nat. Mur.
Impetigo, itching tetter on nape of neck, Nat. Mur.
Inactivity of the skin, Kali. Sulph.
Irritable skin, Nat. Mur.
Jaundiced from biliousness, Nat. Sulph.
Large red blotches, itch violently, Nat. Mur.
Leaden color of face, Nat. Mur.
Leprosy, copper-colored spots, Silica.
Leprosy, nasal ulcerations, Silica.
Lips, eruption on, scabby, smarting pain, Silica.
Lips, lower, vesicles on, Nat. Sulph.
Lips peel off, Kali. Mur.
Lips, pimples on, Kali. Mur.
Lips, upper dry, skin peels off, Nat. Sulph.
Livid skin, Kali. Phos.

Lumps or nodules on face or scalp, Silica.

Lupus, Calc. Phos., Kali. Mur.

Measles, after effects, Kali. Mur.

Measles, hoarse cough, glandular swelling, furred tongue, white or gray deposit, deafness from swelling, Kali. Mur.

Measles in the beginning, and in all stages for heat and fever, Ferr. Phos.; also for inflammatory symptoms of chest, eyes and ears.

Measles, suppressed, with harsh and dry skin, Kali. Sulph.

Measles with excessive secretion of tears and saliva, Nat. Mur.

Nettle-rash after violent exercise or over heating, Nat. Mur.

Nettle-rash over whole body, large red blotches with violent itching, Nat. Mur.

Nettle-rash from indigestion, Kali. Sulph.

Oozing of matter on skin, Calc. Sulph.

Painful and sensitive skin, Nat. Mur., Silica.

Peeling of, Kali. Sulph.

Pimples all over like flea bites, Nat. Phos.

Pimples at puberty, Calc. Sulph., Calc. Phos.

Pimples from heat and congestion, Ferr. Phos.

Pimples, hard, swollen on cheek, Calc. Sulph.

Pimples in region of joints, Calc. Phos.

Pimples like nettle-rash on nape of neck, Silica.

Pimples, matterless under hair, bleeding when scratched, Calc. Sulph.

Pimples on back of hands, itching, Kali. Mur.

Pimples on ear, Calc. Phos.

Pimples on face, Calc. Sulph., Nat. Sulph.

Pimples on scalp, very sensitive, Silica.

Pimples, pustules, scabs, containing pus, Calc. Sulph.

Pimples, sore at opening of right ear, Kali. Phos.

Pimples under beard, Calc. Sulph.

Pimples with mattery scabs on, Calc. Sulph.

Perspiration, acid, sour smelling, Nat. Phos.

Perspiratton excessive about head, Calc. Phos.

Perspiration excessive of feet, Silica.

Perspiration exhausting, heavy odor as during measles, Kali. Phos.

Perspiration, lack of, Kali. Sulph.

Perspiration, offensive of feet or armpits, Silica.

Perspiration on hands from spinal weakness, Calc. Phos.

Perspiration profuse on hands, Silica.

Perspiration suppressed by chill, Silica.

Pruritus of vagina with or without albuminous leucorrhea, Calc. Phos.

Pustules itching, on head and neck, very sensitive, better wrapped warmly, Silica.

Pustules malignant, Kali. Phos.

Pustules on face, Kali. Mur., Silica.

Pustules, painful, Silica.

Rash, like insect bites on arms and legs, running together in large patches, red only when scratched ; prickly feeling all over, Mag. Phos.

Rash on legs and in groups all over, Nat. Mur.

Rash suppressed or receding, with harsh, dry skin, Kali. Sulph.

Rash, with single pimples, Kali. Mur.

Raw skin of little children, Nat. Phos.

Rawness and soreness, smarting, Nat. Mur.

Red face without fever, Nat. Phos.

Redness but no rash, tongue has a burned appearance; produced by excessive use of salt, Nat. Mur.

Red pimples run together, swollen; alkaline fluid oozes out; cuticle comes off in fine scales, itches and stings; better from cold water first, later from warm, Kali. Sulph.

Red spots over whole body, preceded by heat in face, Nat. Mur.

Red spots on face with burning heat, Silica.

Red spots on pit of stomach, Nat. Mur.

Redness of cheeks and gums, heat in face, Nat. Mur.

Rosecolored blotches, brownish white spots, Silica.

Rose rash, Nat. Phos.

Sallow face, Calc. Phos., Ferr. Phos., Nat. Mur. Silica.

Scabs behind ear, Silica.

Scabs between scrotum and right thigh; itching better from scratching; also on forehead, scalp, neck and chest, Nat. Sulph.

Scabs golden yellow, like honey, Nat. Phos.

Scabs greenish, brownish or yellowish, Calc. Sulph.

Scabs greenish, brown or white, forming on pustules, Kali. Mur.

Scabs on ear, thin, cream-like, Nat. Phos.

Scabs on head, Nat. Mur.

Scabby eruption on forehead, just below hair; itching, Nat. Mur.

Scabby eruption on scalp, better in summer, worse toward winter, Silica.

Scalds, when suppurating, Calc. Sulph.

Scald head, Kali. Sulph.

Scald head of children, yellow mattery scabs, Calc. Sulph.

Scalding of scarf-skin, Kali. Sulph.

Scales freely on sticky base, Kali. Sulph.

Scales on scalp, white, no increase of watery secretion, Kali. Mur.

Scales white, floury from blisters, Kali. Mur.

Scalp bald and dry, Kali. Phos.

Scalp, light crust on, in edge of hair like peach gum, Nat. Mur.

Scalp looks raw, as if scalded, Nat. Mur.

Scalp painful, pimples on, with yellow scabs; Calc. Sulph.

Scalp pimples on, painful on combing hair, Nat. Sulph.

Scalp sensitive, sore and tender, Ferr. Phos.

Scalp, suppurations of, discharge yellow and purulent, Calc. Sulph.

Scalp swelling at edge of hair, bleeding when scratched, Calc. Sulph.

Scalp, thin, dry, exfoliated patches on, Silica.

Scalp, yellow crusts on, Calc. Sulph.

Scaly skin in persons of weak constitution, Calc. Fluor.

Scars redden and become painful, Nat. Mur.

Scars following amputation ulcerate, Calc. Phos.

Secretions bloody, watery, Kali. Phos.

Secretions irritate, Kali. Phos.

Secretions sticky, Kali. Mur.

Secretions scurvy, hard infiltrations, Kali. Mur.

Sensitiveness of skin, irritation at root of nose, twitching in corners of eyes, Kali. Mur.

Shingles, Nat. Mur., Kali. Mur.

Skin shines as if greasy, Nat. Mur.

Skin of face cracks, Silica.

Small blisters, Silica.

Small foreign bodies under skin or in larynx, Silica.

Small wounds heal slowly and easily suppurate, Silica.

Small pox, chief remedy, controls formation of pustules, Kali. Mur.

Small pox, heat and fever, Ferr. Phos.

Small pox, pustules discharging, Calc. Sulph.

Small pox, putrid conditions, Kali. Phos.

Small pox, rash suppressed, Kali. Sulph.

Small pox, to promote formation of healthy skin and falling off of crusts, Kali. Sulph.

Small pox with drowsiness or flow of saliva, Nat. Mur.

Sores, discharge pus, unhealthy bad odor, Calc. Sulph., Kali. Phos.

Sores, festers, gatherings, first stage, Ferr. Phos.

Sores or ulcers with whitish or dark gray crusts, Kali. Mur.

Sores with yellow, sticky secretions, discharge thin watery matter, peeling off of surrounding skin, Nat. Mur.

Sores with yellow, watery secretions, effect of ivy poison, Kali. Sulph.

Sore, horny skin, Calc. Fluor.

Sore patches on, Nat. Phos.

Sour sweat on head, Silica.

Sour sweat on head, body nearly dry during first sleep, Silica.

Spots on skin, Nat. Mur.

Stings, insects, Nat. Mur.   Externally also.

Stinging rash over whole body, Nat. Mur.

Thigh, brown spots on inner after syphilis, Nat. Sulph.

Toes, itching, suppurating scabs on toes that have been frozen, Silica.

Tubercles of skin, Calc. Phos.

Unhealthy looking skin, Silica.

Vesicles with bloody contents, Kali. Phos.

Vesicles with colorless, watery contents, Nat. Mur.

Vesicles with watery contents, burst and leave a thin scurf, Nat. Mur.

Wan face, Nat. Mur., Nat. Sulph.

Wax-like skin, tuberculosis, Silica.

Withered, Kali. Phos.

Yellow, brownish, greenish scurfs, Kali. Mur.

Yellow, earthy stain, Silica.

Yellow scabs after breaking of blisters and vesicles, Nat. Sulph.

Yellow scab follows pimples on scalp, Calc. Sulph.

Yollow scales on skin, Nat. Sulph.

Yellowish skin, Calc. Phos., Nat. Sulph., Silica.

TISSUE CELLS.

Abnormal growth on cheek bones, Calc. Fluor.

Abscess about anus, with fistula, Calc. Sulph.

Abscess after spraining toes, Silica.

Abscess bleeds easily after pus forms, Silica.

Abscess deep-seated on bones, Calc. Phos., Kali. Phos., Silica.

Abscess discharges orange-colored fluid through vagina, Kali. Phos.

Abscess discharges unhealthy pus, bloody, ichorous, offensive, dirty, Kali. Phos.

Abscess discharge continues to torpidity of tissues, swelling gone, Calc. Sulph. till healed.

Abscess for inflammation, heat, fever, pain, Ferr. Phos.; if swelling continues alternate with Kali. Mur.

Abscess in second stage, much swelling but no pus, Calc. Sulph., Ferr. Phos., Kali. Mur.

Abscess if suppuration is unavoidable, Silica; after it opens, Calc. Sulph. to heal.

Abscess in upper part of iris, Silica.

Abscess near finger nails, burning, itching, stinging pains, Silica.

Abscess near finger nails when suppuration begins, Calc. Sulph.

Abscess near lumbar region, Silica.

Abscess of breast, much swollen, but no pus formed, Kali. Mur., and apply with vaseline on lint.

Abscess of cornea, Calc. Sulph., Ferr Phos.

Abscess of lips, Silica.

Abscess of lungs, formation of cavities, Silica.

Abscess on inside of thigh, ankle and foot swollen, Silica.

Abscess pelvic, affecting bone, throwing off splinters, Calc. Fluor.

Abscess surrounded by blue border, Nat. Sulph.

Abscess, speedily points, but scanty secretion of pus, Silica.

Abscess to ripen, forming pus, Silica.

Abscess to control suppuration, Calc. Sulph.

Abscess, when there is swelling, Kali. Mur.

All diseases where there is an accumulation of water in the connective tissue, causing watery secretions on skin, Nat. Sulph.

All ailments with swelling of soft parts, threatened suppuration, or discharge of pus and blood, Calc. Sulph.

All obstinate ailments that do not yield to their own remedy, Calc. Phos.

All irritations, congestions and inflammations, caused by excess of blood to any part, Ferr. Phos.

Blister-like sores on lips, ulcerate, ooze bloody matter, Calc. Sulph.

Blistered, sensitive gums, Silica.

Boils, Ferr. Phos., Kali. Mur., Calc. Sulph., Silica.

Boils around eyes or external ear, Silica.

Boils, blood, on cheeks or thighs, Silica.
Boils come in crops, leave indurations, Silica.
Boils, deep-seated, thick, yellow pus, Silica.
Boils for heat, pain, congestion and fever, Ferr. Phos.
Boils for first stage of swelling, Kali. Murr. ; locally also.
Boils or carbuncles, hard, purplish-red, with foul, irritating discharge, Silica.
Boils, small blood boils, Nat. Mur.
Boils, to control suppuration, Calc. Sulph.
Boils, to hasten suppuration, Silica.
Boils, when pus is forming, Silica.
Blows or falls, Ferr. Phos., internally and externally as quick as possible.
Bruises, first remedy, Ferr. Phos.
Bruises, for swelling, Kali. Mur.
Bruises, neglected and threaten to suppurate, Calc. Sulph.
Bunion, Kali. Mur.; also locally; if very hard, Calc. Fluor.

CANCER.

Calc. Sulph. helps cancers, wounds, etc., to heal. Silica causes pus to form and ripens them.
Cancer, discharge thin, yellow, serous, Kali. Sulph.
Cancer, for pain alternate Ferr. Phos. with Kali. Phos. or other indicated remedy.
Cancer in scrofulous constitutions, Calc. Phos.
Cancer of face, Kali. Sulph.
Cancer of lips, Silica.
Cancer of tongue, Nat. Phos., Silica.
Cancer of uterus (womb), Silica.
Cancer on skin, with discharge of thin, yellow matter, Kali. Sulph., internally and externally.

Cancer, painful, offensive discharge, and discoloration, Kali. Sulph.. Kali. Phos.

Canker of mouth and of lips, Kali. Mur.

Canker of mouth, gangrenous, Kali. Phos.

CARBUNCLES.

Carbuncles discharging thick, yellow pus, Silica.

Carbuncles in first stage, for heat, pain, fever and congestion, Ferr. Phos.

Carbuncles in second stage, to control swelling ; alternate Ferr. Phos and Kali. Mur.

Carbuncles on back of neck, Silica.

Carbuncles swelling hard, discolored, purplish-red, ichorous discharge, Silica.

Carbuncle to control suppuration, Calc. Sulph.

Cataract, Calc. Phos., Calc. Fluor., Kali. Sulph., Silica.

Cataract after suppressed foot sweats or eruptions, Silica.

Cataract with weak vision, Calc. Phos.

Constitutional weakness, Calc. Phos. as general tonic.

Convalescence after acute diseases, Calc. Phos.

Cuts and other fresh wounds, bruises and sprains, Ferr. Phos., use locally also.   If swelling continues, Kali. Mur. If suppuration sets in, Calc. Sulph., Silica.   For thin, acrid, fetid discharge or mortification, Kali. Phos.   Proud flesh, Kali. Mur.

Debilitated conditions, with drowsiness, watery vomiting, etc., Nat. Mur.

Development deficient, stunted growth of children, Calc. Phos.

Dropsy, after kidney disease, Calc. Phos.

Dropsy from heart, liver or kidney disease, when other symptoms correspond, Kali. Mur., Nat. Mur.

Dropsy from non-assimilation or anæmia, Calc. Phos.

Dropsy from obstruction of bile ducts and enlargement of liver, Kali. Mur.

Dropsy from weakness of heart or with palpitation, Kali. Mur., Kali Phos.

Dropsy of feet, Nat. Sulph.

Dropsy, post-scarlatinal, if matter forms, Calc. Sulph.

Dropsy with white mucous sediment in urine, Kali. Mur.

Emaciation, even while living well, Nat. Mur.

Emaciation in consumption, Calc. Phos.

Emaciation of neck or feet, Nat. Mur.

Emaciation without apparent ailments, Calc. Phos., Silica.

Face bloated in diphtheria, Nat. Mur.

Face bloated and red, not feverish, Nat. Phos.

Feet slightly swollen and tender, Calc. Sulph.

Fingers puffy, stiff and rigid, Calc. Sulph.

Flat swelling growing on bone of head, Calc. Fluor.

Felon, bone, Silica.

Felon, for heat, pain and fever, Ferr. Phos.

Felon to control formation of pus and promote growth of new nails, Silica.

Fistula on cornea, Silica.

Fistula on anus, with pains in joints in cold, damp weather, Calc. Phos.

Fistula on anus with chest symptoms, Silica.

Fissures of anus, Calc. Phos., Calc. Fluor.

Fissures of anus in children, Calc. Phos.

Fissures of lip, deep and painful, Nat. Mur.

Gathered finger (Whitlow), Calc. Fluor. Locally also. If deep-seated and bone affected, Silica.

Gangrenous conditions, first stage of mortification, Kali. Phos.

Gangrene from perforating ulcer of palate, Silica.

Goitre, chief remedies, Calc. Phos. and Nat. Phos., with others that symptoms call for.

Goitre, for very hard swelling, Calc. Fluor. and Kali. Mur.

Goitre of neck, Calc. Fluor., Nat. Phos., Nat. Sulph.

Goitre, with acid symptoms, tongue yellow or creamy yellow, Nat. Phos.

Goitre, with watery symptoms, tongue very dry, or bubbles of saliva, Nat. Mur.

Granulations around ear, Kali. Mur.

Gum-boils, Silica.

Gum-boils, before suppuration, Kali. Mur.

Gums hot, swollen and inflamed, Ferr. Phos.

Hands, palms of raw and sore and exude watery fluid, Nat. Sulph.

Hang-nails, Nat. Mur., Silica.

Hang-nails, run-arounds, ulcerations, Silica.

Hard, blueish lumps under arm, oozing and scabbing, Calc. Phos.

Head too large, body emaciated, face pale, abdomen hot and bloated, Silica.

Head, lumps on, Calc. Fluor.

Injuries of all kinds ; to prevent pain, congestion, swelling or fever, Ferr. Phos.

Jaws, bony lumps on, Calc. Fluor.

Knee-pan, enlarged sac over, Silica.

Lameness, chronic, from rheumatism of joints, Kali. Mur.

Lameness of rheumatic origin, with shiny, red swelling, Kali. Mur.

Purulent infiltration of tissues after carbuncle, Silica.

Relaxed condition of elastic fibers in general, Calc. Fluor.

Scorbutus (a disease causing bloated countenance, livid spots on skin, foul breath, loose teeth and spongy gums), especially after mercury, Kali. Mur.

Sprains, Ferr. Phos. If swelling remains, Kali. Mur.

Stomach puffed up, Ferr. Phos.

Sty on eye-lid, Ferr. Phos.

Sty in corner of eye, Nat. Mur.

Suppuration, first stage, to control, Calc. Sulph.

Suppuration, to hasten, Silica; after discharging, to heal, Calc. Sulph.

Swelling and suppuration of glands under arms, Nat. Sulph., Silica.

Swelling and soreness of old scars, Silica.

Swelling, erysipelatous on gums and roof of mouth after extraction of teeth, Silica.

Swelling, hard on gums, Nat. Mur.

Swelling, hard on any part, Calc. Fluor.

Swelling, inflammatory of external cavity of ear, Silica.

Swelling of cheeks and gums, painful, Kali. Mur.

Swelling of cheeks with toothache, if suppuration threatens, Calc. Sulph.

Swelling of eustachian tubes, Kali. Sulph.

Swelling of ear, sore, itching and hot, Calc. Phos.

Swelling of face, Calc. Sulph.

Swelling of face with crampy, shooting, darting pains, Mag. Phos.

Swelling of feet and limbs; first soft, then hard, Kali. Mur.

Swelling of feet, Calc. Sulph., Kali. Mur., Nat. Mur., Nat. Sulph.

Swelling of feet to ankles, Silica.

Swelling of fingers, stiffness, Nat. Sulph.

Swelling of fingers, with inflammation, Calc. Sulph.

Swelling of glands around ear, Kali. Mur., Calc. Sulph.

Swelling of glands of neck, Calc. Sulph

Swelling of gums, painful, Kali. Mur.

Swelling of jaw, Silica.

Swelling of limbs, if watery, Nat. Mur.

Swelling of limbs below knee, seem almost bursting, Kali. Mur.

Swelling of lips, after mercury, Kali. Mur.

Swelling of lips hard, painful burning, Calc. Phos., Nat. Mur.

Swelling of lower lip, Kali. Sulph.

Swelling of nose, abscesses, ulcers, etc., Calc. Sulph., Silica

Swelling of parotid glands hard ; suppuration painless if slow, Silica.

Swelling of parotid glands, painful, red after measles, Ferr. Phos.

Swelling of right parotid gland, sore, better in open air, Calc. Sulph.

Swelling of parotid glands in scroflulous persons, Calc. Phos.

Swelling of tympanic cavity, Kali. Sulph.

Swelling of tongue, chronic, Calc.Fluor.

Swelling of tongue, numb, stiff, pimples on, Calc. Phos.

Swelling of tongue, one side, Silica.

Swelling of tongue, dark red, Ferr. Phos.

Swelling red and inflamed after vaccination, Silica.

Swelling scroflulous, Silica.

Swelling soft, Kali. Mur.

Swelling soft, with watery symptoms, Nat. Mur.

Swelling with rheumatism, Kali. Mur.

Syphilis, chronic, Kali. Mur.

Syphilis, chronic, third stage, Calc. Sulph.

Tongue, indurations in, Silica, Calc. Fluor.

Tongue, ringworm on right side of, Nat. Mur.

Tumors, blood, on head, Calc. Fluor.

Tumors, cystic (in a sac) on eyelids, Silica.

Tumors from strain of elastic fibres, Calc. Fluor.

Tumors in left breast, Silica.

Tumors in muscles between ribs, Silica.

Tumors, knots or hardened glands in breast, Calc. Fluor.

Tumors on lower gums, painless, movable, Nat. Sulph.

Tumors, painless, movable on gums, Nat. Sulph.

Tumors, resembling skin on eyelids, Nat. Mur.

Tumors, semi-transparent under tongue (Ranula), Nat. Mur.

Ulcers and spots on cornea, Calc. Phos., Calc. Sulph.

Ulcers around nails, Silica.

Ulcers bleeding easily, Silica.

Ulcers, cancerous, Silica.

Ulcers, coldness in, Silica.

Ulcers discharge thick yellow pus, Calc. Sulph.

Ulcers, edges hard, high and spongy, Silica.

Ulcers, edges callous, Kali. Mur.

Ulcers, fistulous on ankle, Calc. Phos.

Ulcers, fistulous, thick yellow pus, Silica, Calc. Fluor., Calc. Sulph.

Ulcers flat, with bluish, white base, Silica.

Ulcers, follicular on inside of lips, Kali. Mur.

Ulcers from suppuration of membranous parts, Silica.

Ulcers from the use of mercury, Silica.

Ulcers, gray-based on lips, Kali. Mur.

Ulcers in mouth, gray, Kali. Mur.

Ulcers in corners of mouth, Silica.

Ulcers in nose, high up, sensitive to touch, Silica.

Ulcers offensive, bad colored, Kali. Phos.

Ulcers offensive, proud flesh, stinging, burning, itching, Silica.

Ulcers on cheeks, lips, etc., Kali. Mur. ·

Ulcers on cornea, deep, Silica

Ulcers on cornea, perforating or sloughing, Silica.

Ulcers on cornea, scrofulous, Nat. Mur.

Ulcers on cornea, smarting, burning ; feeling as of sand in eyes, Nat. Mur.

Ulcers on eye, sloughing in syphilitic persons ; deep ; discharge profuse ; purulent, Silica.

Ulcers on eye, with sticking, pains in day and night, Silica.

Ulcers on gums, Nat. Mur.

Ulcers on limbs, stitching and burning pain, Silica.

Ulcers, proud flesh in, Kali. Mur., Silica.

Ulcers, scrofulous, slow to heal, Calc. Phos.

Ulcers, stinging, pressing pain in, Silica.

Ulcers with fever. heat and redness, Ferr. Phos.

Ulcers with pale face, Silica.

Ulcers, varicose, Calc. Fluor.

Ulcers, varicose, borders not raised ; not deep nor callous ; worse in wet weather, Nat. Mur.

Ulcers, varicose, just above instep, from injury ; cup-shaped, dark blue, Kali. Sulph.

Ulceration at roots of teeth, Calc. Sulph.

Ulceration of bowels. Calc. Sulph., Nat. Phos.

Ulceration of corners of mouth, itching, Silica.

Ulceration of glands, Calc. Sulph., Silica.

Ulceration of glands, for pain, soreness, redness and heat, Ferr. Phos.

Ulceration of glands with swelling, Kali. Mur.

Ulceration of great toe with stinging pain, Silica.

Ulceration of gums at edges, Kali. Mur.

Ulceration of jaw with swelling, Silica.

Ulceration of limbs, Calc. Sulph.

Ulceration of middle ear, suppuration, foul discharge, Kali. Phos.

Ulceration of mouth of womb, Kali. Mur.

Ulceration of stomach, Nat. Phos.

Ulceration of throat, thick, yellow discharge, Silica.

Ulceration of tongue, Nat. Mur.

Ulceration of tissues, Ferr. Phos.

Ulcerated patches on gums and in throat, putrid, Nat. Mur.

Uneven, hard lumps, Calc. Phos.

Wasting disease (atrophy), with putrid-smelling stools, Kali. Phos.

Warts, Kali. Mur.

Warts in palms of hands, Nat. Mur.

Warts, large, fleshy, suppurating, Silica.

Warts on mouth, Calc. Phos.

Wart-like, raised, red lumps, Nat. Sulph.

Wounds, for inflammation and pain, Ferr. Phos.

Wounds, slow healing, Calc. Sulph.

Wounds, suppurating, Calc. Sulph., Silica.

URINARY ORGANS.

Bed-wetting, with general debility, Calc. Phos., Silica.

Bed-wetting from worms, Nat. Phos.

Bladder, atony (lacking tone) of, Calc. Phos.

Bladder, stone in, to check formation, Calc. Phos.

Bright's disease, Calc. Phos., Kali. Phos.

Bright's disease, for feverish conditions, Ferr. Phos.

Bright's disease, for depressed condition of nerves, sleeplessness, irritability, weary feeling, Kali. Phos.

Diabetes (excessive flow of urine containing sugar or dextrine), chief remedy, Nat. Sulph.

Diabetes, for fevered conditions, Ferr. Phos.

Diabetes, when lungs are involved, Calc. Phos.

Diabetes, with low specific gravity, Nat. Mur.

Diabetes, with nervous weakness, breath peculiar, thirst, emaciation, hunger, Kali. Phos.

Diabetes, with sugary urine, stomach and liver deranged, gray or white tongue, Kali. Mur.

Diabetes, with symptoms of acidity, Nat. Phos.

Diabetes, with voracious hunger from liver disease, Kali. Phos.

Gravel, in bilious persons, Nat. Sulph.

Gravel, sediment in urine, Nat. Sulph., Calc. Phos.

Kidneys, catarrhal inflammation of, Kali. Mur.

Kidneys, diseased after scarlet fever, Ferr. Phos.

Kidneys, gravel, gritty deposit in urine, Calc. Phos.

Urination, constant urging, Ferr. Phos., Silica.

Urination, desire violent, unable to restrain, Nat. Mur.

Urination, desire for, but cannot, Silica.

Urination, discharge involuntary after, Silica.

Urination, discharge glutinous after, Nat. Mur.

Urination frequent, Kali. Phos., Nat. Phos.

Urination frequent in young children, Mag. Phos.

Urination frequent, with great appetite, Kali. Phos.

Urination frequent, burning during, Nat. Phos., Nat. Sulph.

Urination frequent, urging, Calc. Phos.

Urination frequent, urging, with pain in bladder and tip of penis, Ferr. Phos.

Urination, increased desire; pale, watery urine, Nat. Mur.

Urination, increased quantity of urine, Calc. Phos.

Urination, involuntary at night, Silica.

Urination, involuntary when walking, coughing or laughing, Nat. Mur.

Urination, profuse from 8 A. M. to 3 P. M., Calc. Fluor.

Urination scanty, with great urging, Silica, Nat. Phos.

Urination scanty, sluggish stream, few drops retained, Kali. Phos.

Urine, albumen in, Kali. Mur., Kali. Phos., Calc. Phos.

Urine, alkaline, with red sediment, Nat. Mur.

Urine bloody, Nat. Mur., Ferr. Phos.

Urine, brick-dust sediment in, Nat. Mur., Nat. Sulph.

Urine, cannot be passed when others are near, Nat. Mur., Kali. Phos.

Urine dark, like coffee, Nat. Mur.

Urine dark red, with rheumatism, Ferr. Phos.

Urine excessive, watery, Nat. Mur., Ferr. Phos.

Urine, excessive secretion of, Nat. Sulph.

Urine frequently scalding, Kali. Phos., Nat. Phos.

Urine high-colored, Calc. Phos., Ferr. Phos.

Urine high-colored, with feverish smell, Ferr. Phos , Nat. Phos.

Urine, inability to retain, Calc. Phos., Kali. Phos., Nat. Mur., Nat. Phos.

Urine, incontinence of, after a blow on the head, Silica.

Urine, incontinence of, from acidity of stomach, Nat. Phos.

Urine, incontinence of, from paralysis of sphincter, Kali. Phos.

Urine, incontinence of, from weakness of sphincter, Ferr. Phos.

Urine, incontinence of, in the aged, Kali. Phos.

Urine, loaded with bile, Nat. Sulph.

Urine, mucous and pus in after febrile disease, Silica.

Urine, phosphates excessive or deficient, Mag. Phos.

Urine, phosphatic deposits in, Calc. Phos.

Urine, red or saffron color, Kali. Phos.

Urine, red with hectic fever, Calc. Sulph.

Urine, retaining difficult, Calc. Phos., Ferr. Phos., Kali. Phos., Nat. Mur.

Urine, retention of, spasmodic, Mag. Phos.

Urine, retention of, with fever, Ferr. Phos.

Urine, sandy deposit in, clings to side of vessel, Nat. Sulph.

Urine, scanty and dark, Nat. Phos.

Urine, scalding where it touches, Kali. Phos., Nat. Phos.

Urine, spurting of when coughing, Ferr. Phos., Nat. Mur.

Urine, sugary, Kali. Mur.

Urine, suppression or retention of, Ferr. Phos. and Calc. Fluor.

Urine thick, white mucous in, Nat. Mur., Kali. Mur.

Urine, uric acid deposits in, Kali. Mur., Nat. Sulph.

Urine warmer than usual, penetrating odor, Calc. Phos.

Urine, yellow, reddish, sandy deposit in, Kali. Phos., Nat. Sulph.

Urine, voiding large quantities of, with weakness, Calc. Phos.

Urinary organs weak, Silica.

Section 3.—Heat Generation.

The function of heat generation is, from the chemical decomposition of foods and tissues, to maintain a uniform bodily temperature of about 98° in a normal condition.

CHILLS [AGUE].—FEVERS.—INFLAMMATIONS.

AGUE.

Ague, intermittent fever, Nat. Sulph., Nat. Mur. Abstain from rich diet, milk, butter-milk, eggs, fat and fish.

Ague, brought on or made worse by damp weather or moist atmosphere at seashore, Nat. Sulph.

Ague, suppressed by quinine, pain in right side, calves stiff and painful, great pain on motion, skin tawny, Nat. Mur.

Ague, with bilious vomiting, Nat. Sulph.

Ague, with heavy, exhausting sweat, Kali. Phos.

Alternate chills and fever, Nat. Sulph., Nat. Mur.

Alternate chills and heat during day, without sweat, Nat. Mur.

Awakens with chill at night, Nat. Mur.

Chills at evening, cannot get warm in bed, Nat. Sulph.

Chills during courses, towards evening, without thirst, chattering teeth and shaking without external coldness, Nat. Sulph.

Chills in evening, in bed, chilliness frequent, with occasional feverishness, Silica.

Chills every day at same hour, Ferr. Phos.

Chills every other day with severe shaking, Nat. Mur.

Chills followed by heat and sweat, Nat. Sulph.

Chills with spasmodic tightness of breath, Nat. Mur.

Chills while eating, Ferr. Phos.

Chilly in open air or in afternoon, Kali. Mur.

Chilliness all day when moving around, Silica.

Chilliness and goose flesh in afternoon, Nat. Sulph.

Chilliness constant, internal, Silica.

Chilliness constant, and want of animal heat, Nat. Mur., Silica.

Chilliness of whole body, with heat in forehead, pressure at root of nose, thirst, Nat. Mur.

Lower part of body cold, while face is hot, Calc. Phos.

Shivering over back and neck, with warm feet, Kali. Mur.

Shaking chill, outdoors, Calc. Phos.

FEVERS.

Caused by blood poisoning, Kali. Sulph.

Chief remedy in all fevers, Ferr. Phos.; alternate with others called for.

Copious night sweats, Calc. Phos.

Dry heat in evening; hot breath; mouth and tongue dry without thirst; yawning, stretching, Calc. Phos.

Fever with violent heat in head, Silica.

Flushes of heat, Calc. Phos., Nat. Sulph.

Flushes of heat, with headache, Nat. Mur.

Heat and feverishness during any disease. Ferr. Phos.

Heat and pressure on top of head, Nat. Phos.

Heat in ear, Calc. Phos.

Heat in head; red face, vomiting of food, Ferr. Phos., Nat. Mur.

Heat in right ear, in evening, Nat. Sulph.

Heat runs from head down, Calc. Phos.

Heat, redness and swelling of nose, sore pains, worse from blowing nose, Nat. Mur.

Heat, with violent headache and thirst, chilliness over back, sweaty feet, Nat. Mur.

High fever, quick pulse and increased temperature, Ferr. Phos.

Internal coldness, Nat. Sulph.

Increased warmth of body, restlessness, Nat. Sulph.

Purely nervous, fever with high temperature, quick irregular pulse, nervous excitement and weakness, Kali. Phos., Ferr. Phos.

Putrid, camp, farm or brain fever, Kali. Phos.

Sweat easily from exertion, Nat. Mur.

Sweat only on head and face, Silica.

Sweat sour, weakening, Nat. Mur.

Stitches around liver, great languor; emaciation; sallow complexion; urine muddy with red, sandy sediment; loss of appetite, Nat. Mur.

Temperature of body high in disease, Ferr. Phos., Kali. Phos.

To promote perspiration, if not produced by Ferr. Phos., Kali. Sulph.

Typhoid conditions during any fever; twitching, great drowsiness, dry tongue, watery vomiting, Nat. Mur.

Violent fever after confinement, Nat. Sulph.

When temperature rises in evening, Kali. Sulph.

With shivering, hot face and belly-ache, Calc. Phos.

With thirst, dry brown tongue; sleeplessness, unrest, Calc. Fluor.

With thick, white coating on tongue, or constipation, Kali. Mur.

Bilious remittent, Nat. Sulph., Ferr. Phos.

Bilious remittent, with greenish-yellow, or brown or black vomit, Nat. Sulph.

Bilious remittent, with nausea, vomiting, brown coated tongue, yellow skin, constipation or diarrhea, stupor, Nat. Sulph.

Hay fever, Nat. Mur.

Hay fever, watery discharges from eyes and nose, Ferr. Phos., Nat. Mur.

Hay fever, with nervous irritability, Kali. Phos.

Intermittent after the use of quinine, living in damp regions or newly-made grounds, Nat. Mur.

Intermittent, chronic, of children, Calc. Phos.

Intermittent, for fever and vomiting undigested food, Ferr. Phos., Nat. Sulph.

Intermittent, followed by paralysis, Nat. Mur.

Intermittent, great thirst and fever blisters around mouth, Nat. Mur.

Intermittent, in scrofulous children, Calc. Phos.

Intermittent, tongue coated like dry clay, Calc. Sulph.

Intermittent, tongue coated yellow, slimy, Kali. Sulph.

Intermittent, tongue white or grayish white, with fur on back, Kali. Mur.

Intermittent, with acid symptoms, Nat. Phos.

Intermittent, with biliousness, Nat. Sulph.

Intermittent, with cramps in calves; alternate Mag. Phos. and Nat. Sulph.

Intermittent, with debility and profuse perspiration, Kali. Phos.

Intermittent, with vomiting of food, Ferr. Phos.

Intermittent, vomiting of sour, acid masses, Nat. Phos.

Intermittent, when watery symptoms are present, Nat. Mur.

Intermittent, with clear, slimy vomit, like white of egg, Nat. Mur.

Intermittent, with chilliness and habitual feeling of coldness in back, Nat. Mur.

Rheumatic, first and only remedy if taken at once. Ferr. Phos.

Rheumatic, if much swelling, Kali. Mur.

Rheumatic, with shifting, wandering pains, acute or chronic. Kali. Sulph.

Scarlet (Scarlatina), feverish and inflammatory conditions, Ferr. Phos., Kali. Mur. (These two are chief remedies.)

Scarlet, for fever symptoms, Ferr. Phos.

Scarlet, for twitching, Mag. Phos.

Scarlet, for watery vomit, Nat Mur.

Scarlet, putrid condition of throat; typhoidal, Kali. Phos.

Scarlet, rash suppressed, Kali. Sulph.

Scarlet, slight rash, disappearing in twenty-four hours; throat symptoms soon subside, Kali. Mur.

Scarlet, to aid the skin to peel, Kali. Sulph.

Scarlet, with drowsiness, twitching and vomiting of watery phlegm, Nat. Mur.

Scarlet, dry tongue or bubbles of saliva on it, Nat. Mur.

Scarlet, exhaustion, stupor, etc., Kali. Phos.

Scarlet, very light pulse, Ferr. Phos.

Scarlatina, to aid in forming new, healthy skin, Kali. Sulph.

Scarlatina, with swelling of soft palate, Calc. Sulph.

Spotted fever (Cerebro Spinal Meningitis.)

Spotted, as a preventive, Calc. Phos.

Spotted, convalescence slow, Silica.

Spotted, for fever, rapid pulse and delirium, Ferr. Phos.

Spotted, for determination of blood to the head, Nat. Sulph.

Spotted, if stupor or insensibility set in, Kali. Mur.

Typhoid fever, at decline of disease, Calc. Phos. as restorative.

Typhoid, first stage, Ferr. Phos., alternated with Kali. Phos.

Typhoid, brain affections, causing temporary insanity, Kali. Phos.

Typhoid, chilliness, fever, etc., Ferr. Phos.

Typhoid, costiveness, light ochre-colored stools, Kali. Mur., Kali. Phos.

Typhoid, gastric symptoms ; unquenchable thirst ; dry tongue, water tastes spoiled ; nausea after drinking, Nat. Mur.

Typhoid, green, alvine (belonging to the lower belly) discharge, Nat. Sulph.

Typhoid, great debility, profuse sweat ; desire to be magnetized, Silica.

Typhoid, hallucinations of brain, Kali. Phos.

Typhoid, hemorrhage, Ferr. Phos., Kali. Phos., Nat. Mur and enemas of salt water, teaspoonful to a quart.

Typhoid, hemorrhage, clotted and dark, Kali. Mur.

Typhoid, inarticulate speech from dryness of tongue, Kali. Phos.

Typhoid, intestinal ulcers, Calc, Sulph.

Typhoid, malignant symptoms, watery vomiting, dry tongue, twitching, stupor, drowsiness, Nat. Mur.

Typhoid, putrid stools, sleeplessness, offensive breath, weak action of heart, Kali. Phos.

Typhoid, profuse sweat, Silica.

Typhoid, sleeplessness, stupor, delirium, Kali. Phos.

Typhoid, skin dry, with chilly sensation, Kali. Sulph.

Typhoid, to promote rebuilding of tissues, intercur-rently, Calc. Phos.

Typhoid, tongue coated like stale mustard, Kali. Phos.

Typhoid, with haggard face, pulse whizzing or very small, Kali. Phos.

Typhoid, with diarrhea, Calc. Sulph.

Typhoid, tongue white or grayish white with looseness of bowels; light-colored stools, swelling of abdomen, Kali. Mur. If fever, alternate with Ferr. Phos.

Typhoid, secretions around teeth and lips during, Kali. Phos.

Typhoid, wandering in mind with low mutterings; great languor and weakness, Nat. Mur. and Kali. Phos.

Typhoid, with evening aggravations, rise of temperature, rapid pulse, Kali. Sulph.

Typhoid, with constipation, stools light-colored, Kali. Mur.

Typhoid, malignant symptoms, especially of brain, Kali. Phos.

Typhoid, pulse slow, labored, indicating blood poisoning, Kali. Sulph and Kali. Phos.

In the treatment of this fever use rectal injections of hot water freely. If bowels are costive, they prevent the bad results of physic. If diarrhea is present, they cleanse unhealthy membranes.

Yellow fever, chief remedy, Nat. Sulph.

Yellow, feverish or inflammatory conditions, Ferr. Phos.

Yellow, for prostration, Kali. Phos.

Yellow, severe bilious symptoms, greenish yellow, brown or black vomit, Nat. Sulph., alternated with others if required.

Yellow, to prevent, Nat. Sulph., and rectal injections of hot water slightly salted to, thoroughly flush the colon. Also give Ferr. Phos. and Kali. Sulph. in alternation with Nat. Sulph. When perspiration sets in and disease is checked, drop Ferr. Phos. and Nat. Sulph. and give Kali. Mur. and Calc. Phos.

Treat incidental symptoms according to their nature.

INFLAMMATIONS.

Bladder, inflammation of, chronic, Kali. Mur., Ferr. Phos., Calc. Sulph.

Bladder, inflammation of, discharging thick, white, slimy mucous, Kali. Mur.

Bladder, inflammation of, first stage, Ferr. Phos.

Bladder, inflammation of, with prostration, debilitated, Kali. Phos.

Bladder, inflammation of, with pus discharge, Silica.

Bladder, inflammation of, with swelling, Kali. Mur.

Bladder, inflammation of, with violent fever, Ferr. Phos.

Bowels, heat in lower, with green, bilious discharge, Nat. Sulph.

Bowels, inflammation of, Ferr. Phos.

Bowels, inflammation of, second remedy, Kali Mur.

Bones, inflammation of (ostitis), with painful soft parts, Ferr. Phos.

Bones, inflammation of, second stage, Kali. Mur.

Bones, inflammation of membrane of bone (periostitis), Ferr. Phos.

Bones, inflammation of membrane of bone, second stage, Kali. Mur.

Bronchitis (inflammation of bronchi) of young children, Ferr. Phos.

Bronchitis, mucous yellow, slimy, thin, mattery, profuse, Kali. Sulph.

Bronchitis, second stage, when thick phlegm forms, Kali. Mur.

Bronchitis, with heat, fever and pain, Ferr. Phos.

Bronchitis, with white or grayish-white tongue, Kali. Mur.

Cheeks hot, Nat. Mur.   With pain, Ferr. Phos.

Cheeks hot in evening, with chill or other complaint, Calc. Phos.

Congestion of brain, Ferr. Phos.

Congestion of chest, with chilly body, Silica.

Congestion of feet, painful, passive (black and blue), Ferr. Phos.

Congestion of liver, worse when lying on left side, Nat. Sulph.

Congestion of liver, sore, sharp, sticking pains, Nat. Sulph., Ferr. Phos.

Congestion of lungs, bloody-streaked sputa, full, round pulse, Ferr. Phos.

Congestion, with burning, worse in a warm room and after violent exercise, Ferr. Phos.

Conjunctiva, chronic inflammation of, with blister-like granulations on lids, Nat. Sulph.

Conjunctiva, inflammation of, discharge golden-yellow, creamy matter, Nat. Phos.

Conjunctiva, inflammation follicular, Nat. Mur.

Conjunctiva, inflammation scrofulous, with superficial blisters, Kali. Mur.

Conjunctiva, inflammation, with aversion to light, Ferr. Phos.

Conjunctiva, inflammation, with excess of tears, and mucous secretions, Nat. Mur.

Conjunctiva, inflammation, with great dread of light, after measles, Nat. Phos.

Conjunctiva, inflammation, with white mucous secretion, acrid tears, Nat. Mur.

Conjunctiva, inflammation, without suppuration or mucous discharge, Ferr. Phos.

Ears, inflammation, chronic, catarrhal, acrid discharge, Nat. Mur.

Ears, inflammation, chronic, internal or external, Kali. Mur.

Ears, inflammation, from a slap, Calc. Sulph.   .

Ears, inflammation, for fever or pain, Ferr. Phos.

Ears, inflammation of eustachian tubes, Ferr. Phos.

Ears, inflammation of inner ear, after cerebro spinal meningitis, Silica.

· Ears, inflammation, with thick, yellow discharge, Silica.

Ears, inflammation, with thin, bright, yellow secretions, Kali. Sulph.

, Eyes, inflammation of, Ferr. Phos., Nat. Mur., Silica.

Eyes, inflammatian of angles of eye-lids, Calc. Sulph.

Eyes, inflammation of cornea, with thick, yellow discharge, Calc. Sulph.

Eyes, inflammation caused by a wound, Silica.

Eyes, inflammation, dry, Ferr. Phos.

Eyes, inflammation of during dentition, Ferr. Phos.

Eyes, inflammation of, first stage, without mucous or pus, Ferr. Phos.

Eyes, inflammation of, in measles, Ferr. Phos.

Eyes, inflammation of, retina (internal membrane of eye), first stage, Ferr. Phos.

Eyes, inflammation of, retina, third stage, Calc. Sulph.

Eyes, inflammation of, retina, with exudation, Kali. Mur.

Eyes, inflammation of, second stage, when there is discharge of white mucous or yellowish-green matter, Kali. Mur.

Eyes, inflammation of, scrofulous, Nat. Mur., Nat. Phos., .Nat. Sulph.

Eyes, inflammation of, suppurative stage, Calc. Sulph.

Eyes, inflammation of, with excess of tears, Nat. Mur.

Eyes, inflammation of, with discharge of thick, yellow matter, Kali. Sulph.

Eyes, inflammation of, with burning sensation, Ferr. Phos.

Eyes, inflammation of, with superficial blisters, Silica.

Eyes, inflammation of, worse in evening, eyes red, fever, heat, Calc. Sulph.

Eye-lids, inflammation of, aggravated by dampness or drafts, Silica.

Eye-lids, inflammation of, after measles, thick and red, thick discharge, Nat. Mur.

Edges of nostrils inflamed, Silica.

Feet, dry heat in at night, Nat. Sulph.

Feet, hot, Silica.

First stage of all inflammatory diseases, to reduce fever, heat and congestion, Ferr. Phos.

Gums, inflamed, bright red, Ferr. Phos., Kali. Phos.

Gums, inflamed, cheeks swollen, Kali. Mur.

Head, heat and pressure on top during menses, Nat. Sulph.

Head, heat in, hot, red face, vomiting of food, Ferr. Phos., Nat. Mur.

Hips, inflammation of, Ferr. Phos., Kali. Mur., Silica, Calc. Sulph.

Hip-joint, inflammation of, Ferr. Phos., Calc. Sulph., Kali. Mur., Silica.

Inflamed, red swelling after vaccination, Silica.

Inflammation, first stage, heat, redness and pain, Ferr. Phos.

Inflammation, second stage, swelling, or discharge of white mucous, Kali. Mur.

Inflammation, third stage, in all diseases, Kali. Sulph.

Inflammation, third stage, with profuse discharge of

thick, yellow matter, sometimes streaked with blood, Calc. Sulph.

Inflammation and hoarseness from overstrain of voice, Nat. Phos.

Inflammation of membrane of long bone, Silica.

Inflammation of membrane lining the abdomen (peritonitis) Ferr. Phos.

Inflammatory rheumatism, Calc. Phos., Ferr. Phos.

Joints, chronic inflammation, with great swelling and stiffness, Silica.

Joints small, painful inflammation of, worse at night or in bad weather, Calc Phos. and Ferr. Phos.

Kidneys, chronic inflammation of, Calc. Sulph.

Kidneys, heat and tension about, Ferr. Phos.

Kidneys, hot and swollen, Ferr Phos., Kali. Mur.

Kidneys inflamed, first stage, Ferr. Phos.

Kidneys inflamed, second stage, Kali. Mur.

Kidneys inflamed, third stage, Silica.

Knee, chronic inflamation with great swelling and stiffness, Silica.

Knee, inflammation of joint; lancinating pains, Silica.

Knee, inflammation of, after gonorrhea, stiff; worse at night, better from warmth, Silica.

Liver, inflammation of, with slow recovery, Nat. Sulph.

Limbs hot, burn to knees, Nat. Sulph.

Lungs, inflammation of, resulting in suppuration, Silica.

Malignant and gangrenous inflammation, Silica, Kali. Phos.

Nails, inflammation and suppuration about roots of, Nat. Sulph.

Palms, hot in children, Ferr. Phos.

Pharynx, follicular inflammation of, Nat. Mur.

Pharynx. follicular inflammation of, with cheesy lumps, Kali. Mur.

Pharynx, inflammation of, acute, Kali. Mur., Nat. Mur., Silica.

Pharynx, inflammation of, chronic, with constipation, Silica.

Salivary glands, inflammation of, when secreting saliva, Nat. Mur.

Salivary glands, inflammation of, with suppuration, Silica.

Scalp, inflammatory symptoms of, Ferr. Phos.

Skin, inflammation of, for fever and heat, Ferr. Phos.

Skin, inflammation of, with bilious symptoms, Nat. Sulph.

Skin, inflammation of, with swelling, Kali. Mur.

Skin, inflammation of, with yellow, watery exudation, Nat. Sulph.

Skin, inflammation of, with slimy secretions, Kali. Sulph.

Spinal meningitis, Nat. Sulph.

Stomach, acute inflammation, violent pains, distention, vomiting and fever, Ferr. Phos.

Stomach, follicular and ulcerative inflammation, mouth red, Kali. Mur.

Stomach, inflammation of, aggravated by eating, Ferr. Phos.

Stomach, inflammation of, from hot drinks or with white tongue, Kali. Mur.

Stomach, inflammation of, first stage, Ferr. Phos.

Stomach, inflammation of, second stage, Kali. Mur.

Stomach, inflammation of, with failing strength, dry tongue, Kali. Phos.

Stomach, inflammation of, with weakness and debility; nervous prostration, Kali. Phos.

Stomach, inflammation of, with exhaustion, dry tongue, etc., Kali. Phos.

Sunstroke, Nat. Mur

Tongue, inflammation of, dark red, Ferr. Phos., Kali. Mur.

Tongue, inflammation of, with much swelling, Kali. Mur.

Tongue, inflammation of, with exhaustion, Kali. Phos.

Tongue, inflammation of, with suppuration, Silica, Calc. Sulph.

Tonsils, chronic inflammation of, Silica.

Tonsils, inflammation of, acute, Ferr. Phos.

Tonsils, inflammation of, if discharge of pus is impending, Calc. Sulph.

Tonsils, inflammation of, when too late for absorption, Silica.

Tonsils, inflammation of, when suppurating gland will not heal, Silica.

Tonsils, inflammation of, with much swelling, Kali. Mur.

Thighs, inflammation of, double normal size, body emaciated. Silica.

Wind-pipe, inflammation of, Nat. Mur. After inflammation, when pus has begun to form, Silica.

NOTE.—Inflammation, external or internal, treatment the same. Local applications of the remedy should be used where practicable.

SECTION 4.—MOTION AND LOCOMOTION.

The primary function of motion is to make possible cell metamorphosis, then to facilitate nutrition and excretion, and finally to make muscular movements the servants of mind.

BONES.—LIMBS AND JOINTS.—MUSCLES.

BONES.

All diseases of, not caused by injury, Calc. Phos.

All offensive secretions, Silica.

Ankles turn easily, Nat. Mur.

Atrophy (wasting) of, with foul diarrhea, Kali. Phos.

Bow-legs in children, Calc. Phos.; also mechanical supports.

Burning pains in nasal bones, especially at root of nose, Nat. Mur.

Bruised feeling of arm bones, Silica.

Bruised pain in cheek bones when chewing, Nat. Mur.

Bruises on bone surface, with hard, uneven lumps, Calc. Fluor.

Catarrhal affections, when nasal bones are affected with bad odor, Calc. Fluor.

Caries (rotting), painful, Kali. Mur., Silica.

Caries of the long bones or hip joint, Silica.

Diseases, when soft parts are inflamed, hot and painful, Ferr. Phos.

Deficient power of motion, Mag. Phos

Difficulty in moving finger joints, Nat. Mur.

Drawing in shin bones, Calc. Phos.

Drawing, tearing, shooting in hip bone, Calc. Phos.

Ear, bones around ache and hurt, Calc. Phos.

Enlargement of long bones, Silica.

Enlargement of finger bone, Calc. Fluor.

Excrescences on bones, Calc. Fluor.

Exudations from, forming hard, rough, corrugated elevations on bone surface, Calc. Fluor.

Finger bones, swelling of, Calc. Sulph.

Fractures, to aid in uniting, Calc. Phos.; also surgical aid.

Hard swelling on jaw-bones, Calc. Fluor.

Lack of moving power, Kali. Phos.

Necrosis (mortification) of jaw-bones, Silica.

Non-union of after fractures, Calc. Phos.

Of nose, (bones) sore, Silica.

Of nose, affected by disease, Calc. Fluor.

Of spine, affected, Silica.

Rickets, spinal curvature, etc., Calc. Phos.

Soft and friable bones, Calc. Phos.

Spine, curvature of, Calc. Phos.; also proper muscular exercise; mechanical supports if absolutely necessary.

Spine, curvature of to right, sensitive to touch and motion, Silica.

Spine, debility of from exhausting disease, Kali. Phos.

Spine, debility of, with weak legs, Nat. Phos.

Spine, irritation of, paralytic symptoms, cold feet, constipation, Ferr. Phos., Kali. Phos., Nat. Mur.

Spine, oversensitive to pressure or touch; tension and drawing, Nat. Mur.

Spine, partial paralysis from weakness of, Nat. Mur.

Spine, softening of the cord, loss of power, stumbles, Kali. Phos.

Spine, weakness of, Calc. Phos.

Spine, weakness of from sexual excesses, Nat. Mur.

Skull, distention of frontal bone, painful, Silica.

Skull, thin and soft, Kali. Phos.

Ulceration of bones, Calc. Phos., Calc. Sulph., Silica.

Ulceration of jaw-bones, Silica.

Ulceration of bone surface (spina ventosa), Mag. Phos., Calc. Fluor.

Ulceration of bones, with symptoms that call for it, Calc. Sulph.

Ulceration of, with thick, yellow, offensive, mattery discharge, Silica.

Weak and soft bones, Calc. Phos.

LIMBS AND JOINTS.

Ankles, red, swollen, sensitive ; toes burn, Ferr. Phos.

Ankles turn easily, Nat. Mur., Calc. Fluor.

Ankle weak and lame, Nat. Mur., Silica.

Arm and wrist weak, Silica.

Arm, lameness of, falls asleep, Calc. Phos.

Arm heavy, disinclined to move it, Nat. Mur.

Feet, bad odor from without sweat, Silica.

Feet, dislocation, (spontaneous) of the head of long bone, backward, Silica.

Feet give way when walking, Silica.

Feet, veins in distended, Nat. Mur., Ferr. Phos.

Feet weak. Silica.

Hands, no strength in, Nat. Sulph.

Hip-joint disease, first stage, Ferr. Phos.

Hip-joint disease, second stage, when swelling begins, Kali. Mur.

Hip-joint disease, third stage, Calc. Phos.

Hip-joint disease, to control suppuration. Calc. Sulph.

Hip-joint disease, to hasten suppuration, Silica.

Hip-joint disease, when the bone is implicated, Calc. Fluor.

Joints, chronic swelling of, Calc. Phos.

Joints, chronic swelling if scrofulous, Nat. Mur.

Joints, chronic rheumatism of, Nat. Mur., Nat. Phos.

Joints, crackling of, Nat. Phos.

Joints, crackling of, knees stiff; pain in bones, Nat. Sulph.

Joints, dislocated easily. Calc. Fluor.
Joints, elbow, stiffness of, Silica.
Joints, elbow, swelling of, Calc. Fluor and Kali. Mur.
Joints, swelling of, from sprain, much pain, Ferr. Phos.
Joints enlarged, Calc. Fluor.
Joints, gouty enlargements of, Calc. Fluor.
Joints, painful tension under, Nat. Mur.
Joints, rheumatism of with crackling and watery symptoms, Nat. Mur.
Joints, stiffness of, beginning (Ankylosis), Silica.
Joints, swollen, Kali. Mur.
Knee, house-maid's, Calc. Phos., Nat. Mur.
Knee, insipient stiffness of, Silica.
Knee, weak, Nat. Mur.
Limbs, aggravations after rest, Kali. Phos.
Limbs, loss of power in, Nat. Mur.
Limbs, partial paralysis of, after sexual abuse, grief, or outbursts of passion, Nat. Mur.
Limbs, weariness in after walking, Calc. Sulph.
Limbs, weakness of, Calc. Sulph., Silica.
Limbs, weak when descending steps, Silica.
Limbs, weary and exhausted, Nat. Sulph.
Nails, gray, dirty, Silica.
Nails rough, yellow, brittle, Silica.
Toes, gout in, periodcally, Nat. Mur.
Toes, hang-nails with dry skin, Nat. Mur.
Toes, nails ingrowing, Kali. Mur., Silica.

MUSCLES.

Atrophy of, Ferr. Phos., Kali. Mur.
Articulation of jaws, spasmodically closed, Mag. Phos., Silica.
Contraction of in rectum and urethra before urinating, Nat. Mur.

Contraction of muscles in calves, tension in when walking, Silica.

Contraction of in fingers by rheumatism, Ferr. Phos.

Convulsions, limbs stiffened, Mag. Phos.

Convulsive twitching of corners of mouth, Mag. Phos.

Cramps in bowels and wind colic, often with watery diarrhea, Mag. Phos.

Cramps in calves, Mag. Phos., Silica.; inside when walking, Calc. Phos.

Cramps in fingers, Nat. Mur.

Cramps in limbs, Nat. Mur., Mag. Phos., Kali. Mur., Calc. Phos.

Cramps in soles of feet, Silica.

Cramps in stomach, Mag. Phos., Nat. Mur., Silica.

Cramps in stomach, better by tightening clothes, Nat. Mur.

Cramp-like stitching in feet, Nat. Mur.

Debility of muscles in eyes, Nat. Mur.

Distortion of in face, eyes closed, Silica.

Do not contract after using catheter, Mag. Phos.

Involuntary movements of hands, Nat. Mur.

Involuntary shaking of head, Mag. Phos., Kali. Phos.

Jerking of limbs, Nat. Mur.

Jerking of big toe, Calc. Phos.

Jerking of right side and head, Nat. Mur.

Lameness in nates as if beaten, Calc. Phos.

Lock-jaw, Mag. Phos.

Loss of power in muscles, causing contortions and twitchings, Kali. Phos.

Pain in on motion, Silica.

Quivering of in eyelids when reading, Nat. Phos.

Rheumatism of, connected with joints, Ferr. Phos.; Kali. Phos.

Sore muscles in thighs, ham-strings, stiff on rising, cords feel too short, Nat. Phos.

Sore and stiff all over body, Ferr. Phos.

Spasm of neck of bladder, spasmodic stricture, Mag. Phos.

Spasm of bladder or urethra after straining, Mag. Phos., Ferr. Phos., Kali. Phos.

Spasm of eyelids, Calc. Phos., Mag. Phos., Nat. Mur.

Spasm of hands when writing, Silica.

Spasmodic closure of eyelids, Mag. Phos.

Spasmodic twitching of lips, Mag. Phos.

Spasmodic muscular contractions, Mag. Phos.

Squinting, Calc. Phos., Mag. Phos.

Squinting, after diarrhea, Kali. Phos.

Squinting, caused by worms, Nat. Phos.

Stiffness of, Ferr. Phos.

Stiffness of muscles, in neck, from sitting in draft when overheated, Kali. Mur.

Stiffness of, in neck, from cold and dampness, Ferr. Phos., Calc. Phos.

Stiffness of, in neck, head inclined to the right, shoulder raised, Kali. Sulph.

Stiffness of, in neck, with chilliness down back, Silica.

Stiffness of, in neck, with headache, Silica.

Trembling of hands on awaking, Nat. Sulph.

Trembling of hands, shaking, Mag. Phos.

Trembling of hands when writing, Nat. Mur., Nat. Phos., Nat. Sulph.

Trembling of, on left side of face, Kali. Mur.

Twitching of in eyelids, Calc. Sulph, Mag. Phos., Silica.

Twitching of in jaw, Kali. Mur

Twitching of in thigh or limbs, Nat. Mur.

Weakness of in abdomen, Nat. Mur.
Weakness of, can hardly move, Ferr. Phos.

Section 5.—Nutrition.

Nutrition has for its object the supply of wastes.

ABDOMEN.—INDIGESTION.—MOUTH.—STOMACH.—TEETH.
—TONGUE.

ABDOMEN.

Abdomen, bloated, Kali. Sulph., Mag. Phos.
Abdomen, bloated, with watery diarrhea, thirst and colic, Nat. Mur.
Abdomen constantly hard, greatly distended, Silica.
Abdomen distended with gas, Kali. Phos.
Abdomen, grumbling and rolling in, followed by diarrhea, Nat. Sulph.
Abdomen hard, hot, distended, especially in children, Silica.
Abdomen large in children, Calc. Phos., Silica.
Abdomen, motion in as of something alive, Calc. Phos.
Abdomen, much wind in lower part, worse when riding and in evening, Calc. Fluor.
Abdomen, pain in, with diarrhea from change in weather or eating maple sugar, Calc. Sulph.
Abdomen, pressure in after eating, Silica.
Abdomen, rumbling in, loud gurgling, Nat. Mur.
Abdomen, rumbling in, obstinate, Nat. Mur.
Abdomen, rupture of in debilitated persons, Calc. Phos.
Abdomen, rupture of in persons otherwise robust, Ferr. Phos.
Abdomen, soreness in sides of, Calc. Phos.
Abdomen sunken, Calc. Phos., Nat. Mur.

Abdomen swollen, Nat. Mur.
Abdomen tender to touch, Kali. Mur.

INDIGESTION.

Acid risings, Nat. Phos.
Belching, followed by burning in upper abdomen, Calc. Phos.
Belching, hawking, gagging, nausea after breakfast, Calc. Phos.
Belching in afternoon, with nausea, Calc. Phos.
Belching of wind, Mag. Phos.
Belching, with taste of food, Ferr. Phos.
Belching, with vomiting of food, Nat. Mur.
Belching wind, relieves indigestion, Calc. Phos.
Children vomit easily and often, Calc. Phos.
Cold drinks aggravate indigestion, Calc. Phos., Mag. Phos.
Cold drinks relieve indigestion, Ferr. Phos.
Eructations, Silica.
Eructations after eating, nausea, acidity, sleepiness, palpitation, Nat. Mur.
Eructations, alternating with pains in chest and abdomen, Kali. Mur.
Eructations, bitter, or tasteless during day, Nat. Sulph.
Eructations, loud, uncontrollable, with pains in stomach, Silica.
Eructations, offensive after fatty food or milk, Nat. Mur., Kali. Mur.
Eructations relieve colicky pains in stomach, Mag. Phos.
Eructations sour, sour vomiting, acid symptoms, Nat. Phos.
Eructations, with taste of food, Silica.
Eructations, with nausea, Kali. Mur.

Fatty food disagrees, Kali. Mur.

Flatulence, shifting, with distended abdomen, Silica.

Flatulence, with distress about heart, Kali. Phos.

Flatulence, with pains in left side, Kali. Phos.

Flatulence, with sour risings, Nat. Phos.

Flatulence after confinement, Nat. Sulph.

Flatulence before breakfast, collects at night, great pain, Nat. Sulph.

Flatulence, languor, cold feet, no appetite, slow and painful digestion, Silica.

Flatulence, much rolling and rumbling, fixed in right side, Nat. Sulph.

Food aggravates indigestion, distresses, Calc. Phos.

Food causes pain, Nat. Phos.

Food feels like a stone or lead in stomach, Silica.

Food lies in a lump, Calc. Phos.

Fullness and pressure in stomach after eating, Silica.

Indigestion, with griping pains in stomach, Mag. Phos.

Indigestion, with headache, Calc. Phos.

Indigestion, with nervous depression and faint feeling, Kali. Phos.

Indigestion, with pressure and fullness at pit of stomach, water gathers in mouth, Kali. Sulph.

Indigestion, with vomiting of greasy mucous, Kali. Mur.

Indigestion, with watery vomit, Nat. Mur.

Indigestion, worse after eating, Calc. Phos., Ferr. Phos.

Indigestion, worse from sour things, Nat. Phos.

Nausea and vomiting after eating, Ferr. Phos.

Nausea and vomiting of acid fluids and curdled masses (not food), Nat. Phos.

Nausea and vomiting of mucous in morning, Silica.

Pastry disagrees, Kali. Mur.

MOUTH.

Brassy taste of saliva, Kali. Mur.
Creamy yellow coating at back part of roof, Nat. Phos.
Dryness of mouth, without thirst, Silica.
Dryness of mouth, with red gums and thirst, Nat. Sulph.
Dryness of mouth, with or without thirst, Calc. Phos.
Foam at mouth (epilepsy), Silica
Gums bleed easily, Kali. Mur., Kali. Phos., Nat. Mur.
Gums bleed when cleaning teeth, Calc. Sulph.
Gums pale, swollen, soft, bleed easily, Kali. Phos.
Gums red, Nat. Sulph.
Gums spongy, bleeding, mouth sore, Kali. Mur.
Gums spongy, receding, Kali. Phos.
Offensive odor from mouth, Kali. Phos., Silica.
Rawness of mouth, Kali. Mur.
Roof of mouth sore to touch, Nat. Sulph.
Running of saliva, with running of nose, Calc. Phos., Nat. Mur.
Saliva, excess of, Nat. Mur.
Saliva, excess of after meals; Nat. Sulph.
Saliva, profuse, salty, watery, Nat. Mur.
Saliva, tough, stringy, Kali. Mur.
Sore places in mouth, very sensitive, Nat. Mur.
Sore to touch inside, Nat. Sulph.
Sour mouth, with spongy, bleeding gums, Kali. Mur., Nat. Phos.
Syphilitic fur in mouth, Kali. Mur.
Watery froth from mouth, Kali. Mur., Nat. Mur.
Water gathers in mouth, Nat. Mur.

STOMACH.

Anguish in pit of, melancholy, Silica.
Appetite excessive, Calc. Sulph., Kali. Mur., Nat. Mur., Nat. Phos., Silica.

Appetite excessive, and thirst, Calc. Sulph.

Appetite excessive, with fullness after taking little, Nat. Mur.

Appetite not satisfied, Kali. Phos.

Appetite slight, Nat. Sulph.

Aversion to bread, Nat. Mur., Nat. Phos., Nat. Sulph.

Aversion to coffee, Nat. Mur.

Aversion to milk, Ferr. Phos.

Aversion to warm, cooked food, Silica.

Cold food or drink causes diarrhea, Nat. Sulph.

Desires only cold things, Silica.

Desires only sweet things, Kali. Phos.

Desires tea, green, sour vegetables, fruit, Calc. Sulph.

Desire for ice or ice-cold water, Nat. Sulph.

Desire for strong-tasting things, beer, alcohol, etc., Nat. Phos.

Dread of hot drinks, Kali. Sulph.

Dyspepsia, Calc. Phos., Ferr. Phos., Kali. Mur., Kali. Phos., Kali. Sulph., Nat. Mur., Nat. Phos., Silica.

Hungry soon after eating, from weakness or nervousness, Kali. Phos.

Longing for beer, Nat. Mur., Nat. Phos., Nat. Sulph.

Longing for bitter things, Nat. Mur.

Longing for salt, oysters, fish, meal, sour things, Nat. Mur.

Morning sickness, Nat. Phos.

Nausea after eating, Silica, Nat. Mur.

Nausea, constant, Nat. Sulph.

Nausea after exercise that raises bodily heat, Silica.

Nausea after drinking, Nat. Mur.

Nausea after stools, Silica.

Nausea from smoking, or drinking coffee, Calc. Phos.

Nausea immediately after eating, heaviness of head, bitter eructations, Nat. Mur., Nat. Sulph.

Nausea, with faintness and headache, Calc. Fluor.

Nausea, with headache, pains in stomach, vertigo, Calc. Sulph.

Nausea, with pain in pelvis, Calc. Sulph.

Nausea, with sour risings, Nat. Phos.

Nausea, with violent palpitation, Silica.

Qualmishness before meals, Nat. Sulph.

Relaxation of stomach, Calc Phos.

Secretion of lactic acid excessive, Nat. Phos.

Sickness, deathly, sudden, Ferr. Phos.

Stomach flabby, relaxed, Calc. Phos.

Stomach trouble, eyes large and projecting, Kali. Mur.

Stomach trouble, scanty but normal stools, Nat. Sulph.

Sourness of stomach, vomited matter sets teeth on edge, Ferr. Phos., Nat. Phos.

Stomach tender to touch, Ferr. Phos.

Thirstlessness, Kali. Phos.

Thirst and appetite excessive, Calc. Sulph.

Thirst constant, without desire to drink, Nat. Sulph.

Thirst for much water, Ferr. Phos.

Thirst violent, unquenchable, Kali. Phos., Nat. Mur.

Vomiting after nursing, Silica.

Vomiting after cold drinks, Calc. Phos.

Vomiting followed by waterbrash, Calc. Phos., Silica.

Vomiting from stomach-ache, Mag. Phos.

Vomiting in morning, with great exhaustion, Silica.

Vomiting in morning before eating, Ferr. Phos.

Vomiting of bile, Nat. Mur., Nat. Sulph.

Vomiting of blood, Ferr. Phos , Kali. Mur.

Vomiting of curdled masses, Nat. Phos.

Vomiting of dark substances, like coffee-grounds, Nat. Mur., Nat. Phos.

Vomiting of food, Nat. Mur.

Vomiting of greenish water, Nat. Sulph.

Vomiting of sour fluids, Nat. Mur., Nat. Phos.

Vomiting of tenacious phlegm, Silica.

Vomiting of undigested food, Calc. Fluor., Ferr. Phos.

Vomiting of white slime, Kali. Mur.

Vomiting, preceded by dizziness, Nat. Sulph.

Vomiting, with pains, Ferr. Phos.

Vomiting, with trembling hands, Calc. Phos.

Waterbrash, heart-burn and acidity, Nat. Phos.

Waterbrash, without acidity, Nat. Mur.

Waterbrash, with brown tongue, chilliness or nausea, Silica.

Weak, gone feeling at pit of stomach, Kali. Phos.

Weakness of stomach, by spells, Nat. Mur.

TEETH.

Teeth, chattering of, nervous, Kali. Phos.

Teeth, children grind during sleep, Nat. Phos.

Teeth, decay of too rapid, Calc. Phos., Calc. Fluor.

Teeth, dulness of, Calc. Fluor.

Teeth, enamel of brittle, deficient, Calc. Fluor.

Teeth, enamel of rough and thin, Calc. Fluor.

Teeth loose, Nat. Mur., Silica.

Teeth, molar, right lower, decayed, tender, and sensitive to cold air and water, Calc. Sulph.

TONGUE.

The tongue aids in determining the condition of the digestive organs, the mucous membranes, the blood, and the nervous system.

In some acute and chronic diseases there are no tongue

signs nor symptoms.   The following, when present, are good indications for the use of the Salts:

Brown, Kali. Phos., Kali. Sulph., Nat. Sulph.

Creamy, Nat. Phos.

Dry, Calc. Phos., Kali. Mur., Kali. Phos., Nat. Mur.

Frothy, Nat. Mur.

Furred, natural color, Ferr. Phos., Kali. Mur., Kali. Sulph., Nat. Phos., Nat. Sulph.

Flabby, Calc. Sulph.

Gray, Kali. Mur., Nat. Sulph.

Green, Nat. Sulph.

Red, Ferr. Phos., Kali. Mur., Kali. Phos , Mag. Phos., Nat. Sulph.

Slimy, Kali. Mur., Kali. Sulph., Nat. Mur., Nat. Sulph.

White, Calc. Phos., Kali. Mur., Kali. Phos., Kali. Sulph.

Yellow, Calc. Sulph., Kali. Sulph., Nat. Phos.

Indurated, Calc. Fluor., Silica.

Pale, Calc. Phos., Ferr. Phos., Nat. Mur.

Tremulous, Kali. Phos., Mag. Phos.

Swollen, Kali. Mur., Calc. Fluor.

Ulcers, Kali. Phos., Kali. Mur., Nat. Mur., Silica.

Bitter taste, Nat. Sulph., Kali. Mur., Calc. Phos.

Sour taste, Nat. Phos., Calc. Sulph., Silica.

—T. M. Triplett, M. D.

Tongue, broad, pallid, puffy ; pasty coating, Nat. Mur.

Tongue, bubbles of frothy saliva on edges, Nat. Mur.

Tongue, burning on tip of, Calc. Phos., Nat. Mur., Nat. Sulph.

Tongue, center of dark brown, Nat. Phos.

Tongue, clean and red, Ferr. Phos.

Tongue, clean and moist, excessive saliva, Nat. Mur.

Tongue, coating clear, slimy, watery, Nat. Mur.

Tongue, coating curdy, bitter, Nat. Sulph.

Tongue, coating brownish mucous, Silica.

Tongue, coating dirty greenish gray or brownish green, Nat. Sulph.

Tongue, coating heavy, white, Kali. Mur.

Tongue, coating creamy yellow, Nat. Phos.

Tongue, coating grayish white, Kali. Mur.

Tongue, brownish, mustard colored, Kali. Phos.

Tongue, coating thin, white, not mucous, Kali. Mur.

Tongue, coating white fur at root, worse in morning, Calc. Phos.

Tongue, coat white fur of syphilitic origin, Kali. Mur.

Tongue, coat yellow at base, Calc. Sulph., Nat. Phos.

Tongue, cracked appearance of, Calc. Fluor.

Tongue, dark red and inflamed, Ferr. Phos.

Tongue, dry, white, without fever, Kali. Mur.

Tongue, dry in morning, Kali. Phos.

Tongue, dryish or slimy, Kali. Mur., Kali. Sulph.

Tongue, eruptions on from sea bathing, Nat. Mur.

Tongue, excessive dryness in morning, Kali. Phos., Nat. Mur.

Tongue, hardening of, Silica.

Tongue, heavy, difficult speech, Nat. Mur., Calc. Phos.

Tongue, mapped, Nat. Mur., Calc. Fluor.

Tongue, numbness of, Calc. Phos.

Tongue, one side feels numb and stiff, Nat. Mur.

Tongue, red, pain without exudation, Ferr. Phos.

Tongue, seamed with a deep red line, Calc. Sulph.

Tongue, stiffness of, Calc. Phos., Nat. Mur.

Tongue, talking difficult, Kali. Mur., Calc. Phos.

Tongue, watery froth from, Nat. Mur.

SECTION 6.—REPRODUCTION.

FEMALE SEXUAL ORGANS.—MALE SEXUAL ORGANS.—PREG-
NANCY.—PARTURITION.—INFANCY.

FEMALE SEXUAL ORGANS.

Abdomen, weight and fullness in, Kali. Sulph.

Abscess, discharging orange-colored fluid through the vagina, Kali. Phos.

Amenorrhea (retention or delay of the flow), depression, lassitude, debility, Kali. Phos.

Amenorrhea, with suppressed foot-sweats, pain in abdomen, Silica.

Bearing-down feeling, Calc. Fluor.

Breasts, cancer of, Silica.

Breasts, gathered, Kali. Mur.

Breasts, hard knots or lumps in, Calc. Fluor. and Silica.

Breasts, inflammation of, hardening, suppuration, fistulous ulcers, thin, watery, offensive discharge, Silica.

Breasts, inflammation of, to prevent matter forming, Calc. Sulph.

Breasts, inflammation of, with persistent hardness, Calc. Fluor.

Breasts, inflammation of, with pus discharge, Silica., Calc. Sulph.

Breasts, inflammation of, with unhealthy, offensive pus, Kali. Phos.

Breasts, nodular, knotty tumors of, Silica.

Bladder, aching in neck of, prostration, Calc. Phos.

Chlorosis (a disease caused by suppression of menses), Ferr. Phos., Nat. Mur.

Coition (sexual intercourse), aversion to, Nat. Mur.

Coition, burning, smarting in vagina during, Nat. Mur.

Coition, easy and light hearted after at first ; later, ill humored, Nat. Mur.

Coition, nausea during, Silica.

Coition, painful from dryness of vagina, Nat. Mur., Ferr. Phos.

Coition, prevented by painful, spasmodic contraction of the sphincter vaginæ muscle, Ferr. Phos., Mag. Phos.

Clitoris (a small glandiform body resembling the structure of the male penis), erect after urination, with sexual desire, Calc. Phos.

Discharge, bloody between periods, Silica.

Discharge, deep red or blackish red, Kali. Phos.

Discharge, scalding, smarting, Nat. Mur.

Discharge, sickening or sour smelling, Nat. Phos.

Discharge, thin, with offensive odor, Kali. Phos.

Dragging in groin or small of back, Calc. Fluor.

Dysmenorrhea (difficult and painful menstruation), face red, pulse faster, excessive congestion, Ferr. Phos. before periods as a preventive. Alternated with Kali. Phos. and occasional doses of Calc. Phos. it is almost a specific. Drink freely of hot water. For excessive crampy pain, Mag. Phos. Use locally also by dissolving in hot water and applying on cloths over uterus.

Dysmenorrhea, with convulsions. Mag. Phos.

Flushes of heat, Calc. Phos., Nat. Sulph.

Drawing pain over pubes, with discharge of blood, and followed by earache, Calc. Phos.

Genitals, external, itching of, Nat. Mur., Silica.

Genitals, feel as if filling with blood, Calc. Phos.

Genitals, pimples on Mons Veneris, Nat. Mur.

Genitals, pressure or other sensations over, Calc. Phos.

Genitals, pressing and pushing towards in morning, Nat. Mur.

Genitals, pressure and pain in, with leucorrhea, Calc. Phos.

Genitals, string felt between uterus and sacrum, sensitive to touch, Nat. Mur.

Genital, stitching all through womb and pelvis, Kali. Phos.

Genitals, throbbing, stinging, tickling, sore aching in, Calc. Phos.

Gonorrhea.   (See Male Sexual Organs).

Growling in stomach and aching legs, as if menses would begin, Kali. Phos.

Hysteric fits of crying, Kali. Phos.

Labia (the lips), aching, warm feeling between, Calc. Phos.

Labia, inner, stitching pains in, Calc. Phos.

Leucorrhea (whites), Calc. Phos. intercurrently as constitutional tonic.

Leucorrhea, acrid, obstinate, Kali. Mur., Nat. Mur.

Leucorrhea, acrid, greenish, Nat. Mur., Kali. Sulph.

Leucorrhea, acrid, profuse, corrosive, Nat. Sulph., Silica.

Leucorrhea, acrid, watery, Nat. Phos.

Leucorrhea, after child-birth, Nat. Sulph.

Leucorrhea, before menses, Nat. Mur.

Leucorrhea, causes biting pains, Silica.

Leucorrhea, causes hair to fall from pubes, Nat. Mur.

Leucorrhea, causes itching of pudendum, Nat. Mur.

Leucorrhea, causes rawness and itching, Nat. Phos.

Leucorrhea, creamy or honey colored, Nat. Phos.

Leucorrhea, cream-like discharge passes unconsciously afternoons, Calc. Phos.

Leucorrhea, excoriating, tenacious, yellow, Silica.

Leucorrhea, excoriating, tetter-like, Nat. Mur.

Leucorrhea, greenish, especially after walking, Nat. Mur., Kali. Sulph.

Leucorrhea, increases as menses decrease, Calc. Phos.

Leucorrhea, in gushes, Silica.

Leucorrhea, in morning, transparent and watery, Nat. Mur.

Leucorrhea, in young women who have been crossed in love, Calc. Phos.

Leucorrhea, like white of egg, day and night, Calc. Phos.

Leucorrhea, mild, white, not transparent, Kali. Mur.

Leucorrhea, preceded by colic and bearing down, Nat. Mur.

Leucorrhea, scalding, acrid, Nat. Mur. Kali. Phos.

Leucorrhea, thick, yellow, bloody, Calc. Sulph.

Leucorrhea, tearing upward from right side to navel, anxiety, better when leucorrhea appears, Calc. Phos.

Leucorrhea, very profuse, with excessive debility, Nat. Mur.

Leucorrhea, watery, slimy, smarting, accompanied by dull, heavy headache, Nat. Mur.

Leucorrhea, while urinating, Silica.

Leucorrhea, yellow before menses, Nat. Mur.

Leucorrhea, yellowish green, blistering, too short menses, Kali. Phos.

Leucorrhea, yellowish, watery, mattery, Kali. Sulph.

Note.—Daily injections of hot water containing the indicated remedy should be used in all cases of leucorrhea. Remove the cause, if possible.

Listlessness, Calc. Phos.

Menses, acrid, profuse, corrosive, Nat. Sulph., Silica.

Menses, afternoon headache over eyes during, Nat. Phos.

Menses, anxious, sad, before, Nat. Mur.

Menses, backache during and after, Calc. Phos.

Menses, bearing down during, Calc. Fluor.

Menses, before, bloody saliva, Nat. Mur.

Menses, before, burning, tearing, cutting pains, Nat. Mur.

Menses, before, eyelids twitch, eyes heavy, Nat. Mur.

Menses, before, disposition to faint, Nat. Mur.

Menses, before, fatigue, Kali. Phos.

Menses, before, feels as if vulva was enlarged, sore perineum, Silica.

Menses, before, great sexual desire, Calc. Phos.

Menses, before, griping, rumbling in bowels, Calc. Phos.

Menses, before, irritable, squamish, sad, anxious, Nat. Mur.

Menses, before, lassitude and trembling, Nat. Mur.

Menses, before, nose-bleed, Nat. Sulph.

Menses, before, nymphomania, organs erect, desire insatiable, Calc. Phos.

Menses, before, nausea, sweet morning eructations, Nat. Mur.

Menses, before, palpitation, Nat. Mur., Kali. Phos.

Menses, before, pressing pain in forehead, Silica., Nat. Mur.

Menses, before, scraping face-ache, Nat. Mur.

Menses, before, sleepiness and leucorrhea, Calc. Phos.

Menses, before, sore, burning in vagina, Nat. Mur.

Menses, before, soreness of wrists, Nat. Phos.

Menses, before, toothache, Nat. Mur.

Menses, bitter taste at beginning of, Calc. Phos., Nat. Sulph.

Menses, black and clotted, Calc. Phos., Kali. Mur.

Menses, black red, Kali. Phos.

Menses, bloated feeling during, Kali. Phos.

Menses, blood rushes to head during, Calc. Phos.

Menses, breasts swell and suppurate, Kali. Phos., Calc. Sulph.

Menses, burning and soreness of vulva during, Silica.

Menses, burning of palate during, Nat. Sulph.

Menses, bright flow in young girls, Calc. Phos.

Menses, cold extremities during, Calc. Phos., Ferr. Phos.

Menses, constipation before or during, Silica., Nat. Mur.

Menses, crampy pains in lower part of abdomen during, Mag. Phos.

Menses, dark, especially in rheumatic subjects, Calc. Phos.

Menses, delayed or suppressed, Kali. Mur., Kali. Phos., Nat. Mur.

Menses, delayed, in young girls, Nat. Mur.

Menses, delayed, with heated face, heavy abdomen, bloody saliva, Nat. Mur., Ferr. Phos.

Menses, digging in abdomen during, followed by thirst, Nat. Sulph.

Menses, drawing between shoulders during, Silica.

Menses, drawing, pressing, sore as if should come, Calc. Phos.

Menses, diminished, like white of egg, worse in morning and increased, with white stool of bad odor, Calc. Phos.

Menses, dryness of vagina, and aversion to coitus after, Nat. Mur.

Menses, during lactation, Calc. Phos.

Menses, eruption on inner thighs during, Silica.

Menses, every three weeks, Ferr. Phos., Kali. Sulph., Nat. Mur.

Menses, every three weeks, with pressure in abdomen and back, Ferr. Phos.

Menses, every two weeks, black and clotted, Calc. Phos., Kali. Mur.

Menses, excessive, dark, clotted, or tough, tarry, Kali. Mur.

Menses, excessive, with bearing-down pains, Calc. Fluor.

Menses, feet cold days and burn nights, during, Nat. Mur.

Menses, flow freely when walking, Nat. Sulph.

Menses, followed by congestion of head, Ferr. Phos.

Menses, followed by headache, Nat. Mur.

Menses, followed by increasing throbbing headache, Calc. Phos.

Menses, followed by itching in vulva, Nat. Mur.

Menses, followed by lassitude and trembling, headaches, twitching and weakness worse, Calc. Sulph.

Menses, followed by sensation as if cords of knees were shortened, Nat. Phos.

Menses, followed by want of appetite, Calc. Phos.

Menses, fullness in abdomen during, Kali. Sulph.

Menses, morning headache, dull, heavy, Nat. Mur.

Menses, headache, dull, bursting, Kali. Phos.

Menses, headache three to seven days before, or just before, Calc. Phos., Nat. Mur.

Menses, inflammation about heart, with scant flow, Nat. Mur.

Menses, irregular, every two or three months, Silica.

Menses, irregular, scant, almost black, first day thick, Kali. Phos.

Menses, labor-like pains before and during, Calc. Phos., Mag. Phos.

Menses, languor, with diarrhea and leucorrhea during, Calc. Phos.

Menses, last too long, Kali. Phos., Kali. Mur., Nat. Mur.

Menses, loss of appetite before and during, Calc. Phos.

Menses, limbs heavy, fatigue, diarrhea, backache, shooting pains, weary all over, Calc. Phos.

Menses, melancholy, anxiety, weary of life during, Silica., Kali. Phos.

Menses, more flow at night, Nat. Mur.

Menses, obscured sight, and toothache, during, Silica.

Menses, painful, flushed face, quick pulse, bright-red blood, Ferr. Phos.

Menses, pain in left leg and groin during, Kali. Phos.

Menses, pain in abdomen during, Silica.

Menses, pain severe, crampy, before or during, Mag. Phos.

Menses, pale, thin, watery, Nat. Mur., Nat. Phos.

Menses, premature and profuse in nervous subjects, Kali. Phos.

Menses, pressure over pubes during, Calc. Phos.

Menses, preceded by violent colic, shuddering, acrid leucorrhea, Silica.

Menses, preceded by sweet eructations in morning, Nat. Mur.

Menses, pressure in small of back during; every three weeks, Ferr. Phos.

Menses, retention or delay of flow, depression, nerve debility, Kali. Phos.

Menses, red face, much pain, pulse accelerated, Ferr. Phos.

Menses, retarded, scant, with colic, Nat.Sulph.

Menses, scant a day or two, then profuse, Nat. Mur.

Menses, scant and delayed, with debility, Nat. Mur.

Menses, scant, with knotty stools streaked with blood, Nat. Sulph.

Menses, scant, with inflammation about heart, Nat. Mur.

Menses, sensation as of heavy lump in anus during, Silica.

Menses, stomach grumbles during, Kali. Phos.

Menses, sore and burning vulva, Silica.

Menses, strong-smelling, acrid, Silica.

Menses, strong sexual desire before, followed by free flow, Calc. Phos.

Menses, stitching pains in left side of head before or during, Calc. Phos.

Menses, sadness, colic, headache, palpitation during, Nat. Mur.

Menses, severe pain on top of head during, Ferr. Phos.

Menses, suppressed from bathing, followed by epileptic spasms, Calc. Phos.

Menses, suppressed from putting feet in cold water, debility, headache and backache, Nat. Mur.

Menses, stitching from loins into uterus before, Nat. Mur.

Menses, too early, Calc. Phos., Kali. Mur., Nat. Mur. Kali. Phos.

Menses, too early and too scanty, Kali. Phos., Silica.

Menses, too early and too scanty, with dragging in left lower jaw, Silica.

Menses, too early, with bright blood, Calc. Phos.

Menses, too early, with dark blood, Kali. Mur.

Menses, too pale, afternoon headache over eyes, Nat. Mur.

Menses, too late and too scanty, or too early and too profuse, Nat. Mur.

Menses, too late, acrid, makes thighs sore, Nat. Sulph.
Menses, too late and profuse, Silica.
Menses, too late and dark, or light and then dark, Calc. Phos.
Menses, too profuse, with heavy odor, Kali. Phos.
Menses, thin, not coagulating, Kali. Phos.
Menses, tearing pain in tibia during, Silica.
Menses, tired, sleepy during, Kali. Phos.
Menses, toothache and obscured sight during, Silica.
Menses, twitchings during, Calc. Sulph., Mag. Phos.
Menses, vertigo and throbbing in forehead during, Calc. Phos.
Menses, weakness during, Calc. Sulph.
Menses, white water instead of, Silica.
Menses, whites, and sleepiness during the day before, Calc. Phos.
Menstrual colic before or during flow, Mag. Phos.
Menstrual colic in sensitive, pale, irritable people, Kali. Phos.
Menstrual colic, with quickened pulse, red face, Ferr. Phos.
Metorrhagia (hemorrhage of the womb), Silica., Ferr. Phos.
Metorrhagia, from standing in cold water, Silica.
Metorrhagia, with offensive foot-sweat, icy body, painful hemorrhoids, Silica.
Nipples, inflammation of, crack and suppurate, Silica., Calc. Fluor.
Ovarian region, dull pain in, with bearing down in uterus, Ferr. Phos., Calc. Fluor.
Ovarian region, pain in, extending down thighs, Nat. Mur.
Ovaries, inflammation of, Ferr. Phos.

Ovaries, neuralgia of, darting like lightning, worse on right side, Mag. Phos.

Ovaries, pain in, Kali. Phos.

Prolapsus, uterine, aching back, better when lying on it, cutting in urethra after urinating, Nat. Mur.

Prolapsus, in debilitated persons, Calc. Phos.

Pain and soreness across abdomen to right side, Kali. Phos.

Pain, drawing from right to left over pubes, with discharge of blood, and followed by earache, Calc. Phos.

Pain, from right groin to left hip, Calc. Phos.

Pudenda (genital organs as a whole), itching of, Silica.

Pudenda, burning and soreness of during menses, Silica.

Sacrum (posterior bone of pelvis), intense pain across, Kali. Phos.

Sexual desire, diminished, Kali. Phos., Nat. Mur.

Sexual desire, increased, Calc. Phos., Kali. Phos., Silica.

Sexual desire, increased after menses, Kali. Phos.

Sexual desire, increased after urination, Calc. Phos.

Sexual desire, increased, with pressing in uterus, Calc. Phos.

Sexual desire, increased, with feeling of pulse in all parts of the body, Calc. Phos.

Sexual desire, insatiable before menses, Calc. Phos.

Sexual desire, insatiable from plethora or spinal irritation, Silica.

Sterility, Nat. Mur., Silica.

Sterility, due to acid secretions, Nat. Phos.

Uterus, aching in, in the morning, Calc. Phos.

Uterus, bearing down of, with constant dull pain in either ovarian region, Ferr. Phos., Calc. Fluor.

Uterus, cancer of, Silica.

Uterus, cramps of, cutting and burning in loins, Nat. Mur., Mag. Phos.

Uterus, cutting pains in through to backbone, Calc. Phos.

Uterus, distress and weakness in region of, Calc. Phos., Nat. Phos.

Uterus, distress and weakness, worse at stool and urination, Calc. Phos.

Uterus, displacement of, Calc. Fluor., Calc. Phos., Kali. Phos.

Uterus, dragging pain in region of, and in thighs, Calc. Fluor.

Uterus, glassy phlegm from, obstinate constipation, Nat. Mur., Calc. Phos.

Uterus, hard, like stone, Calc. Fluor.

Uterus, hemorrhage from, Kali. Mur. Ferr., Phos.

Uterus, inflammation of, Ferr. Phos.

Uterus, inflammation of the cellular tissues, Silica.

Uterus, neck of, hardened, Silica.

Uterus, neck of, red, swollen, shot-like pouches to the touch, Calc. Phos.

Uterus, pressing down, must sit to prevent prolapsus, Nat. Mur., Calc. Fluor.

Uterus, painful, swollen, thickened, ulcers on, Nat. Mur., Kali. Mur.

Uterus, polypus of, Calc. Phos.

Uterus, prolapsus of, with aching lumbar region, better lying on back, Nat. Mur.

Uterus, prolapsus of, from myelitis, Silica.

Uterus, prolapsus of, with sinking feeling after stool, Nat. Phos.

Uterus, prolapsus of, worse during stool and menses, Calc. Phos.

Uterus, relaxed and flabby, Calc. Fluor.

Uterus, rheumatic pains, with displacements, Nat. Phos , Calc. Fluor.

Uterus, soreness and pressure in ; also in loins ; heat flushes, Calc. Phos.

Uterus, sour-smelling, acid discharge from, Nat. Phos.

Uterus, stitching from loins into before menses, Nat. Mur.

Uterus, ulceration of mouth and neck, Silica.

Vagina, aching in after nose-bleed, Calc. Phos.

Vagina, burning in, like fire up into chest, pains both sides of bladder and uterus, Calc. Phos.

Vagina, burning and soreness in after urinating, Nat. Mur.

Vagina, coolness, paleness or dryness of, Nat. Mur.

Vagina, dryness in 'after menses, Nat. Mur.

Vagina, inflammation of, Ferr. Phos.

Vagina, pains from navel drawing to, Calc. Phos.

Vagina, pains in, with flushes and faintness, Calc. Phos., Kali. Phos.

Vagina, pressing down feeling in, Silica.

Vagina, sore, aching, or burning in, before menses, Nat. Mur.

Vagina, soreness, aching, pressure and heat flushes, Calc. Phos.

Vagina, serous cysts in, Silica.

Vagina, swelling of, on awakening, Calc. Phos.

Vagina, weakness of, after urinating, Nat. Mur.

Vagina, smarting of, after urinating, Nat. Mur.

Vulva, burning and sore during menses, Silica.

Vulva, itching of, Nat. Mur., Silica.

Vulva, inflammation of, Nat. Mur., Nat. Sulph.

Vulva, inflammation of, with falling of the hair, Nat. Mur.

Vulva, sensation as if enlarged before menses, Silica.

Vulva, worms in, Silica.

Vulva, swelling of, on awakening, Calc. Phos.

Weakness of organs, Calc. Phos.

MALE SEXUAL ORGANS.

Albuminous discharge from urethra, Calc. Phos.

Bubo (an inflamed gland), suppurating, soft swelling, Kali. Mur.

Bubo, with purulent discharge, Calc. Sulph.

Chancre (a sore from syphilitic poison), Kali. Mur. and Nat. Mur. alternately ; Kali. Mur. locally, also.

Chancre, hard, Calc. Fluor. internally and externally.

Chancre, malignant, spreading, with sloughing surface, Kali. Phos.

Chancre, soft, Kali. Mur.

Coition, bruised feeling over body after, Silica.

Coition, burning and itching at opening, after, Nat. Phos.

Coition, prostration and weak vision after, Kali. Phos.

Coition, sensation in right side of head, as if paralyzed, after it ; also sore limbs, Silica.

Desire, absent or increased, Nat. Mur.

Desire, diminished, apathy and chilliness, Kali. Mur.

Desire, irregular, Nat. Phos.

Desire, morning or evening, with erections, Nat. Sulph.

Desire, very weak, Silica.

Desire, with frequent erections and emissions, Nat. Mur.

Desire, without erections, Nat. Phos.

Desire, with physical weakness, Nat. Mur.

Discharge of prostatic fluid, Nat. Mur.

Discharge, yellow, slimy, gleet, Kali. Sulph.

Dropsy of scrotum and prepuce, Nat. Sulph., Nat. Mur., Ferr. Phos.

Dropsy of testicles, Calc. Fluor., Calc. Phos., Nat. Sulph., Nat. Mur.

Emissions, at night, prostration afterward, Silica.

Emissions, after masturbation, depression, aching sacrum, sweating scrotum, worse before emission, better after, Silica.

Emissions, every night, Nat. Mur., Nat. Phos.

Emissions, every night, first with dreams, later without sensation, Nat. Phos.

Emissions, followed by chilliness and lassitude, and increased desire, Nat. Mur.

Emissions, followed by pain through right groin, Nat. Phos.

Emissions, retarded, Nat. Mur.

Emissions, soon after coition, Nat. Mur.

Emissions, without erections, Kali. Phos.

Emissions, with erections and itching scrotum, Kali. Mur.

Emissions, without dreams or sensation, Nat. Phos.

Emissions, weak back and trembling limbs after, Nat. Phos.

Erections, in morning, without sexual excitement, Nat. Mur.

Erections, painful, with downward curvature of penis in gonorrhea, Kali. Mur.

Erections, rigid in morning, painful, Silica.

Erections, while riding in a carriage, without desire, Calc. Phos.

Erections, without sexual desire, Silica.

Eruptions, itching, moist or dry, Silica.

Genitals, bad odor from, Nat. Mur.

Genitals, itching of, burning after scratching, Nat. Sulph.

Genitals, weak feeling in, Nat. Mur.

Glands, of groin, painful but not swollen, Nat. Mur.

Glans penis, crawling and itching of, Nat. Mur.

Glans penis, pus-like matter on, Nat. Mur.

Glans penis, red spots on, Silica.

Gonorrhea (gleet), Kali. Mur.

Gonorrhea, chronic, in debilitated persons, Calc. Phos.

Gonorrhea, chronic, thick, yellow discharge, Silica.

Gonorrhea, discharge, clear or greenish, itching, Nat. Mur.

Gonorrhea, discharge, thick, white or yellowish-white, swelling, Kali. Mur.

Gonorrhea, discharge, of blood, Kali. Phos.

Gonorrhea, discharge, of blood and pus, or purulent matter, Calc. Sulph.

Gonorrhea, discharge, watery, transparent, Nat. Mur.

Gonorrhea, discharge, watery, scalding, Calc. Phos., Nat. Mur.

Gonorrhea, discharge, slimy, yellow or greenish, Kali, Sulph.

Gonorrhea, discharge, yellowish-green, thick, enlarged prostate, Nat. Sulph.

Gonorrhea, from acrid leucorrhea or menses, yellow or black discharge, Nat. Mur.

Gonorrhea, inflammatory stage, Ferr. Phos.

Gonorrhea, of long standing, thick, fetid pus, chilly feeling, Silica.

Gonorrhea, of glans or urethra, with chordee, Kali. Mur.

Gonorrhea, of glans or urethra, with purulent, yellow or greenish mucous discharge, Kali. Sulph.

Gonorrhea, pus-like, bloody discharge, shreddy, Silica.

Gonorrhea, suppurative stage, Calc. Sulph.

Gonorrhea, suppressed, Nat. Sulph.

Gonorrhea, thick, fetid pus, worse after sweating, Silica.

Gonorrhea, to destroy injurious effects of nitrate of silver, Nat. Mur.

Hair, loss of from pubes, Nat. Mur.

Herpes, moist, sore, itching between thighs and scrotum, Nat. Mur.

Hydrocele (dropsy within testicle), Silica, Calc. Phos., Nat. Mur., Nat. Sulph.

Hydrocele, in children, Kali. Mur.

Impotence, spermatorrhea, spinal irritation, poor digestion, Nat. Mur , Calc. Sulph.

Irritability, of sexual organs, excessive, Nat. Phos.

Lascivious thoughts and dreams, Silica.

Masturbation (self abuse), Calc. Phos.

Penis and testicles, hot at height of a chill, Silica.

Penis and testicles, swollen, Silica, Kali. Mur.

Penis, discharge, of clear mucous, watery slime, sometimes yellowish, Nat Mur.

Penis, discharge, of thin liquid, burning and itching, Nat. Mur.

Penis, discharge, of prostatic fluid, without erections, when thinking of sexual things, Nat. Mur.

Penis, discharge, of prostatic fluid when straining at stool, Silica.

Penis, discharge, purulent, yellow or greenish pus, Kali. Sulph.

Penis, discharge, pus, or pus-like, may be bloody, Silica.

Penis, discharge, slightly shreddy, Silica.

Penis, discharge, yellow or black, Nat. Mur.

Penis, discharge, yellowish-green, thick, little pain, Nat. Sulph.

Penis, discharge, yellow, purulent, spots linen, pain in urination and in glands of groin, not swollen, Nat. Mur.

Penis, shooting pain in tip, and in bladder, Calc. Phos.

Penis, shooting pains from perineum, Calc. Phos.

Penis, sharp, pricking pains in, Silica.

Physical weakness after excesses; even paralysis, Nat. Mur.

Prostate gland, abscess of, suppurative, Calc. Sulph.

Prepuce, itching and red, Silica.

Prepuce, retracted behind glands, Nat. Mur.

Prostate, irritated or inflamed, Ferr. Phos.

Prostate, enlarged, no pain, but hardening, Silica, Calc. Fluor.

Prostate, enlarged, pus and mucous in urine, Nat. Sulph.

Prostatitis, thick, fetid pus from urethra, Silica.

Pus and mucous in urine, Nat. Sulph.

Relaxation and weakness after urinating, Calc. Phos.

Scrotum, itches, Calc. Phos., Silica.

Scrotum, itches, and disturbs sleep, Nat. Mur.

Scrotum, itching of, sweating, sore, pimples on, Calc. Phos.

Scrotum, oozing of fluid from, Calc. Phos.

Scrotum, relaxed, flabby, Nat. Mur., Calc. Phos.

Scrotum, sweating of, Calc. Phos., Silica.

Semen, escapes in urine, Calc. Phos., Nat. Phos.

Semen, smells like stale urine, Nat. Phos.

Semen, thin, watery, Nat. Phos.

Spermatorrhea, Calc. Sulph., Kali. Mur., Kali. Phos., Nat. Mur., Nat. Phos., Silica.

Spermatorrhea, with impotency, Calc. Sulph., Nat. Mur.

Syphilis, chronic, Calc. Sulph., Kali. Mur., Silica., Nat. Mur., Nat. Sulph.

Syphilis, chronic, with suppurations and hardening, Silica.

Syphilis, with evening aggravations, Kali. Sulph.

Syphilis, with serous discharge, Nat. Mur.

Syphilis, with white discharge, Kali. Mur.

Testicles, aching in after suppressed mumps or gonorrhea, Nat. Mur.

Testicles, cold and clammy, Calc. Phos.

Testicles, induration (hardening) of, Calc. Fluor., Silica.

Testicles, inflammation of, Ferr. Phos., Calc. Phos.

Testicles, inflammation of, from suppressed gonorrhea, Kali. Mur., Kali. Sulph.

Testicles, squeezing pain in, Silica.

Testicles, swelling of, Calc. Phos., Silica.

Testicles, wasted, Calc. Phos., Nat. Mur.

Urethra, burning and itching in after coitus, Nat. Phos.

Urethra, burning in after urinating, Nat. Mur.

Urethra, burning in, with painful erections, especially in evening, Calc. Phos.

Urethra, itching in, Kali. Mur.

Urethra, sore on pressure, Nat. Mur.

Ulcer, syphilitic, Kali. Phos.

Varicocele, Ferr. Phos.

Weak feeling in sexual organs after stool, Calc. Phos.

PREGNANCY.

Abortion, threatened, Kali. Mur , Silica.

Aching, in limbs, during pregnancy, Calc. Phos.

Aching, in navel region, extending to sacral, Calc. Phos.

Bitter taste during pregnancy, Nat Sulph.

Brain function perverted during pregnancy, Kali. Phos., Kali. Mur.

Breasts, burning and pain in, Calc. Phos.
Breasts, burning and pain in, prevent sleep, Silica.
Breasts, feel large and sore to touch, Calc. Phos.
Breasts, fissures and ulcers of, Silica.
Breasts, fistulous ulcers after abscess, Silica.
Breasts, hard lumps in (if Kali. Mur. fails), Silica.
Breasts, hard lumps or knots in, Calc. Fluor.
Breasts, inflamed, Ferr. Phos., Calc. Phos., Kali. Mur., Kali. Phos., Silica.
Breasts, inflamed, first stage, for fever, Ferr. Phos.
Breasts, inflamed, for swelling before pus forms, Kali. Mur.
Breasts, inflamed, after pus forms, Silica.
Breasts, inflamed, with brown, dirty, offensive discharge, Kali. Phos.
Breasts, inflamed, with suppuration, Calc. Sulph., Silica.
Breasts, itching and swollen, Silica.
Breasts, itching, bad-colored, bad-smelling, gangrenous pus, Kali. Phos.
Breasts, itching, deep red in center, swollen, hard, sensitive to touch, high fever, Ferr. Phos., Silica.
Breasts, sore to touch, Calc. Phos.
Breasts, ulcers of, discharge serum or milk, Silica.
Congestion, of chest, and palpitation during, Nat. Mur.
Convulsions, during, Mag. Phos.
Cough, during, Ferr. Phos., Nat. Mur.
Cough, during, with ejection of urine, Ferr. Phos.
Debility, of vital power, during, Kali. Phos.
Decline, before or after child-birth, Calc. Phos.
Desire, for salt or salty food, during, Nat. Mur.
Discharge, bloody, during, Kali. Phos.
Eructations, of food, during, Ferr. Phos.

Faint, gone feeling in stomach, during, Nat. Mur., Kali. Phos.

Headache, during third month of, Ferr. Phos.

Heavy weight on pelvis, pressing down, and backache, Kali. Phos.

Heartburn, during, Nat. Mur.

Heartburn and palpitation, Nat. Mur.

Heartburn, up into throat, Calc. Phos.

Hemorrhage, during, Calc. Fluor.

Hemorrhage, after abortion, worse by motion, or from mental or sexual excitement, Silica.

Hungry, without appetite, during, Nat. Mur.

Languor, during, Calc. Phos.

Mania, during, Kali. Mur , Kali. Phos.

Miscarriage, in weak subjects, Kali. Phos.

Miscarriage, flooding, to tone up contractile power of womb, Calc. Fluor.

Morning sickness, Kali. Mur., Nat. Mur., Nat. Phos.

Morning sickness, with vomiting of food, Ferr. Phos.

Morning sickness, with vomiting frothy, watery phlegm, Nat. Mur.

Morning sickness, with vomiting bilious fluids, Nat. Sulph.

Morning sickness, with vomiting sour masses or fluids, Nat. Phos.

Morning sickness, with vomiting white phlegm, Kali. Mur.

Morning sickness, with diarrhea, with yellow, slimy, watery and purulent discharge, Kali. Sulph.

Motions of child too violent, between third and ninth months, Silica.

Nausea, during, Nat. Mur.

Nausea, with sour risings, Nat. Phos.

Night-pains, during, Kali. Phos.
Nipples, cancer or hard tumor of, Silica.
Nipples, darting, burning in, Silica.
Nipples, drawn in like a funnel, Silica.
Nipples, inflamed, ulcerated, Silica.
Nipples, sore and ache, Calc. Phos., Ferr. Phos.
Piles, during, Nat. Mur.
Quivering, in lower abdomen, front, during, Calc. Phos.
Sore feet and lameness, during, Silica.
Soreness of right groin, during, Calc. Phos.
Urine, contains albumen, during, Kali. Mur., Nat. Mur.
Urine, escape of, during, Ferr. Phos., Nat. Mur.
Urine, excessive, during, Nat. Mur.
Urine, painful and difficult, Nat. Mur.
Waterbrash, constant, during, Nat. Mur.
Weariness, in limbs, during, Calc. Phos.

PARTURITION.

Kali. Phos., occasional doses a month before labor, gives tone and vigor to system, and makes labor easier and safer.

After delivery, Ferr. Phos., followed or accompanied by indicated remedies. Use also, in water, to syringe vagina night and morning.

After-pains, felt in hips, Silica
After-pains, too weak, contractions too feeble, Calc. Fluor.

Breasts, broken, before formation of pus, Kali. Mur.
Breasts, broken, when pus begins to form, Calc. Sulph.
Breasts, sharp pains in, when nursing, Silica.
Child-bed, fever, Ferr. Phos., Kali. Phos., Kali. Mur. Use douche of Ferr. Phos., thirty grains to a quart of hot water.

Child-bed, fever, aching near navel, and extending to lower back, worse in forenoon, Calc. Phos.

Child-bed, fever, at the beginning, alternate Ferr. Phos. and Kali. Mur. very frequently ; Ferr. Phos. to control inflammation, and Kali. Mur., swelling.

Child-bed, fever, for brain symptoms and blood poison, Kali. Phos.

Child-bed, fever, for second stage, Kali. Phos.

Child-bed, fever, mania and absurd notions in, Kali. Phos.

Convulsions, during birth, Mag. Phos., Nat. Mur.

Discharge, following delivery, suppressed, boring pains in temple and nerve above orbit of eye, Silica.

Labor-pains, feeble, ineffectual, spurious, Kali. Phos.

Labor-pains, progress slowly, pains feeble, seemingly from sad feelings and gloomy forebodings, Nat. Mur.

Labor-pains, spasmodic, cramps in legs, Mag. Phos.

Labor-pains, spasmodic convulsions, excessive expulsive effort, Mag. Phos.

Labor-pains, tedious, from weakness, Kali. Phos.

Lacerations, Ferr. Phos. internally and externally.

Menstruation, during lactation (nursing), Calc. Phos.

Milk, changeable, alkaline to neutral or acid, watery and thin, Calc. Phos.

Milk, failure of, or scanty supply, Calc. Fluor.

Milk-leg (inflammation of veins of leg and thigh, usually following birth, characterized by cord-like hardness and tenderness of affected vein, followed by swelling of limb), Nat. Sulph.

Milk, salty, Nat. Mur.

Milk, suppressed, Silica.

Milk, spoiled, salty and blueish ; child refuses, Calc. Phos.

Milk, watery, Nat. Mur., Calc. Phos.

Several weeks after confinement, prostration, restlessness, sleeplessness, bad taste, loss of appetite, thirst, red tongue, headache, inflammation and eruption in vulva, Nat Sulph.

Sharp pains, in breast or uterus (womb) while nursing, pain in back, discharge which follows delivery increased, Silica.

INFANCY.

Birth-marks (nævi), Ferr. Phos.

Blood-tumor, of cranial region (Cephalhoematoma), Calc. Fluor.

Child, has sore mouth and fever, Nat. Mur., Ferr. Phos.

Child, has flabby scrotum and chills, Nat. Mur.

Child, refuses food, Nat. Mur.

Child, vomits often and easily, Calc. Phos.

Child, vomits if it nurses, Silica.

Child, wants to nurse constantly, Calc. Phos.

Colic, with drawing up of legs, Mag. Phos.

Colic, with worms, green, sour-smelling stools, vomiting curdled milk, Nat. Phos.

Convulsions, from teething, without fever, Mag. Phos. and Calc. Phos., alternately.

Convulsions, with fever, Ferr. Phos.

Delicate, pale appearance when breeding second teeth, Calc. Phos.

Diaper, reddish yellow, Calc. Phos.

Fontanelles, closure of, delayed, Calc. Phos.

Fontanelles, reopening of, Calc. Phos.

Infantlle paralysis, recent, Kali. Phos. ; if connected with teething, Calc. Phos. also.

Skull, flat swelling on, Calc. Fluor.

Slow, in learning to walk, Calc. Phos., Nat. Mur.

Teething, cold tumors and emaciation during, Calc. Phos.

Teething, cramps, with fever, during, Ferr. Phos.

Teething, cramps, without fever, during, Mag. Phos. and Calc. Phos.

Teething, difficult and painful, Calc. Phos., Silica.

Teething, dribbling of saliva, during, Nat. Mur.

Teething, eyes inflamed, dry, during, Ferr. Phos., Calc. Phos.

Teething, feverishness, during, Ferr. Phos.

Teething, gums inflamed, Ferr. Phos.

Teething, slowness of, Calc. Phos., Silica.

Teething, spasm of bladder, during, Mag. Phos.

Teething, spasm of glottis, during, Mag. Phos.

Teething, spasmodic cough, during, Mag. Phos.

Teething, too late, Calc. Phos.

Thrush (sore mouth), Ferr. Phos.

Thrush, with flow of saliva, Nat. Mur.

SECTION .7.—RESPIRATION.

The function of respiration is to take in oxygen and water for the use of the system, and carry off the wastes that have been taken up by the carbonic acid and water that are thrown off with the exhaled air.

BRONCHIAL TUBES AND THROAT.—CHEST AND LUNGS.— NOSE.

BRONCHIAL TUBES AND THROAT.

Breathing, cannot take a deep breath, Silica.

Breathing, constant desire to draw deep breath, Nat. Sulph.

Breathing, difficult, as if epiglottis was nearly closed, Calc. Fluor.

Breathing, difficult, as from taking cold, Calc. Fluor.

Breathing, difficult, cannot lie down or stoop, Silica.

Breathing, difficult, in damp, rainy weather, Nat. Sulph.

Breathing, difficult, on ascending steps, Kali. Phos., Nat. Mur.

Breathing, difficult, only during a storm, Silica.

Breathing, difficult, till 10 P. M., better lying down, worse getting up, Calc. Phos.

Breathing, difficult, when coughing, Silica.

Breathing, difficult, when lying on back, stooping or running, Silica.

Breathing, difficult, with contraction of chest, Calc. Phos.

Breathing, difficult, worse when sitting up, Calc. Phos.

Breathing, easier in open air, Nat. Mur.

Breathing, deep, causes stitches in right side, later in left, Nat. Sulph.

Breathing, deep, causes pleuritic stitches, Ferr. Phos.

Breathing, desire to breathe deeply and sigh, pain in chest, shooting in liver, Calc. Phos.

Breathing, gives jerking pain in back, and shooting in left breast and temple, Calc. Phos.

Breathing, more frequent, short and difficult, Calc. Phos.

Breathing, oppressed, in young girls, with suppression of menses, Nat. Mur.

Breathing, oppressed, wheezing, anxious, Nat. Mur.

Breathing, short and oppressive, Ferr. Phos.

Breathing, short, on walking fast, Nat. Mur., Nat. Sulph.

Breathing, short, with cough, Calc. Phos.

Breathing, short, with constipation, and tendency to chronic disease, Calc. Sulph.

Breathing, short, with pain in small spot on coughing, Calc. Phos.

Breathing, short, with piercing pain in left side, Nat. Sulph.

Breathing, suffocative, Calc. Phos., Calc. Sulph., Nat. Mur.

Breathing, suffocative attacks, after great dryness of mouth, eyes protrude, loss of consciousness, Calc. Sulph.

Breathing, so difficult eyes protrude, must open doors and windows, only during thunder storms, Nat. Sulph.

Breathing, with deep sighing, Silica.

Breath, hot, Nat. Mur.

Breath, offensive, in diphtheria, and ulceration, Kali. Mur., Kali. Phos.

Breath, offensive, inflammation of stomach, Kali. Phos.

Bronchi, affections of, in rickety children, copious expectoration, Silica.

Bronchi, asthmatic, yellow mucous raised easily, Kali. Sulph.

Bronchi, rattling in, much mucous in throat, Nat. Mur.

Bronchi, rough and sore, Silica.

Clergyman's sore throat, Calc. Phos., intercurrently; acute, at commencement, Ferr. Phos.

Cough, acute, short, spasmodic, very painful, Ferr. Phos.

Cough, acute, short, like whooping-cough, Kali. Mur.

Cough, awakens at night, Silica.

Cough, better from warm drinks, Silica.

Cough, causes bursting pain in head, Nat. Mur.

Cough, causes cutting and stinging in chest, Nat. Mur.

Cough, causes pain in bronchi and wind-pipe, Kali. Phos.

Cough, causes patient to hold chest, Nat. Sulph.

Cough, causes stitches in chest, Calc. Phos.

Cough, croupy, hard, with white tongue, Kali. Mur.

Cough, dry and scratching, after dinner, Kali. Phos.

Cough, dry, hacking, during pregnancy, with spurting urine, Ferr. Phos.

Cough, dry, hard, with soreness from cold, no expectoration, Ferr. Phos.

Cough, dry, tickling, yellow or bloody sputa, Nat. Mur.

Cough, excited by empty swallowing, Nat. Mur.

Cough, excited by tickling in throat, Kali. Phos., Nat. Mur., Silica.

Cough, exudations cause soreness and chafing, Nat. Sulph.

Cough, from elongated palate, Nat. Mur., and gargle of sumach tea.

Cough, from bronchial tickling, Ferr. Phos.

Cough, from irritated wind-pipe, Ferr. Phos.; with scanty, thick, yellowish-white phlegm, Kali Phos.

Cough, from 6 A. M. to 6 P. M., Calc. Phos.

Cough, from tickling throat at night, Kali. Phos.

Cough, from tickling throat, later lower down, then in chest, explosive during day, Silica.

Cough, from tickling throat, or pit of stomach, Nat. Mur.

Cough, hacking, Calc. Fluor., Ferr. Phos., Nat. Mur., Silica.

Cough, hacking, after dinner, from tickling in throat, not relieved by coughing, Calc. Fluor.

Cough, hacking, caused by tickling in throat, Silica.

Cough, hacking, in morning, with hoarseness and sore throat, Calc. Phos.

Cough, hard, rough at night, Kali. Mur.

Cough, hollow, spasmodic, Silica.

Cough, hard, hoarse, croupy, with weariness in upper throat, Kali. Sulph.

Cough, hard, with protruding eyes, Kali. Mur.

Cough, incessant, with difficult breathing, Kali. Mur., Ferr. Phos.

Cough, influenza, with difficult hearing, ringing in ears, Silica.

Cough, irritation, seated in region of stomach, Nat. Mur.

Cough, laryngeal, morning, on rising, tough, tenacious expectoration, Silica.

Cough, loose, at night, Silica.

Cough, loud, barking, fever, restlessness at night, dry heat, great oppression, Ferr. Phos., Kali. Phos.

Cough, noisy, protruding eyes, itching anus, Kali. Mur.

Cough, paroxysmal, Mag. Phos.

Cough, paroxysmal, worse at night, or during day when asleep, Ferr. Phos.

Cough, preceded by pressure in throat, Kali. Phos.

Cough, rattling or whistling, green or soap-suds expectoration, Kali. Phos., Nat. Mur.

Cough, rough, short, hacking, breathless, Nat. Mur

Cough, sequel to intermittent, Nat. Mur.

Cough, short, obstinate, Nat. Mur.

Cough, spasmodic, at night, no expectoration, Mag. Phos.

Cough, spasmodic, in morning, when dressing, worse in open air, Ferr. Phos.

Cough, spasmodic, suffocative in bed, serous, frothy expectoration, Nat. Mur.

Cough, spasmodic, with involuntary urination, Ferr. Phos., Nat. Mur.

Cough, short, painful, with soreness of lungs, Ferr. Phos.

Cough, shocks in region of stomach, during, Nat. Mur.

Cough, sour food aggravates, Nat. Phos.

Cough, tickling, in evening, Calc. Phos.

Cough, violent, with nasal catarrh, Kali. Mur.

Cough, tickling, on walking, or deep inspiration, Nat. Mur.

Cough, with catching of breath, Nat. Mur.

Cough, with cutting, tearing, in chest, Nat. Mur.

Cough, with dry chest and throat, as from sulphur, Kali. Mur., Nat. Mur.

Cough, with excess of tears, saliva, etc., Nat. Mur.

Cough, with fever, dryness and thirst, Calc. Phos.

Cough, with hawking phlegm, in morning, Nat. Mur.

Cough, with hoarseness, Calc. Phos., Kali. Phos., Silica.

Cough, with hectic fever, Calc. Sulph.

Cough, with leucorrhea, Nat. Mur.

Cough, with loss of breath or palpitation, Nat. Mur.

Cough, with nose-bleed, during menses, Nat. Sulph.

Cough, with pain in throat, chest, testicles, and spermatic cord, Nat. Mur.

Cough, with profuse, purulent, thick expectoration, and soreness of chest, Silica.

Cough, with retching and vomiting, Nat. Mur.

Cough, sore throat, and expectoration of small, bad-tasting lumps, Silica.

Cough, with scanty, mucous expectoration, Silica.

Cough, whooping, Mag. Phos.

Cough, without expectoration, Ferr. Phos., Kali Phos., Mag. Phos.

Cough, winter cough, with watery symptoms, Nat. Mur.

Cough, when bending head or touching larynx. Ferr. Phos.

Cough, when sitting erect, Nat. Mur.

Cough, worse from air of room, exercise or rapid motion, Nat. Mur.

Cough, worse from cold drinks, in evening, lying down or in morning, Silica.

Cough, worse in cold, damp, rainy weather, Nat. Sulph.

Croup, Calc. Sulph., Ferr. Phos., Kali. Mur., Kali. Phos., Nat. Mur.

Croup, last stage, extreme weakness, pale or livid, Kali. Phos.

Croup, membranous, Kali. Mur.

Croup, violent fever at outset, Ferr. Phos.

Diphtheria, bad effects from, amaurosis (blindness), Silica.

Diphtheria, cough, difficult breathing, chest constricted, watery froth from mouth, excessive urination, Nat. Mur.

Diphtheria, face puffy, pale, heavy drowsiness, watery stools, much saliva or vomit of watery fluid, dry tongue, swelling of glands, burning throat and mapped tongue, Nat. Mur.

Diphtheria, involving the larynx, Kali. Mur.

Diphtheria, gray ulcers, tough, stringy mucous, nose-bleed, ravenous hunger, followed by loss of appetite, dry, painful throat, difficult swallowing, hoarse voice, Kali. Mur.

Diphtheria, putrid, very offensive odor, gangrenous, Kali. Phos.

Diphtheria, extends into wind-pipe, Calc. Phos. alternated with Calc. Fluor.

Diphtheritis, of soft palate, Calc. Sulph.

Larynx, dry, Calc. Fluor., Nat. Mur.

Larynx, dry, hoarse toward night, no cough, Calc. Phos.

Larynx, dry catarrh of, yellow or bloody sputa, hoarse, oppressed, Kali. Mur.

Larynx, fibrous, painless swelling of, and of thyroid cartilage, Silica, Kali. Mur.

Larynx, foreign bodies in, Silica.

Larynx, roughness and hoarseness of, Silica.

Laryngismus Stridulus, (spasmodic croup), constricted chest, stiff limbs, Mag. Phos.

Larynx, raw and sore, from coughing, Nat. Mur.

Lungs, hemorrhage from, Ferr. Phos., Kali. Mur. and Silica.

Palate, diphtheria of the soft, tonsils much swollen, Calc. Sulph., Kali. Mur.

Palate, elongated, Nat. Mur., Calc. Fluor.

Palate, sore, yellow, pale, Silica.

Palate, swollen, Silica, Kali. Mur.

Pharynx (region of the throat behind nose, mouth and larynx), catarrh of, white exudation, Kali. Mur.

Pharynx, red and sore, tonsils also, Ferr. Phos., Calc. Sulph.

Quinsy, periodical, Silica.

Swallowing, difficult, Kali. Mur.

Swallowing, difficult, as from paralysis, Silica.

Swallowing, difficult, can only swallow liquids, Nat. Mur.

Swallowing, empty more painful than of food or drink, Nat. Mur.

Swallowing, food passes over a sore spot, Nat. Mur.

Swallowing, food goes down wrong way, or seems to lodge in throat, Nat. Mur.

Swallowing, solids ejected, with gagging and suffocation, Nat. Mur.

Swallowing, soreness on left side of throat, Silica.

Throat, acute, sore, with white points at opening of gland ducts, Kali. Mur.

Throat, ailing, with acid stomach, Nat. Phos.

Throat, better from warm drinks, Calc. Fluor., Calc. Phos.

Throat, better when swallowing food, Nat. Phos.

Throat, choke easily when swallowing, Silica.

Throat, constricted, stitches and swelling, Nat. Mur.

Throat, dryness and pain in, Kali. Mur., Silica.

Throat, dryness in at night, Calc. Phos.

Throat, dryness of, violent cough, Kali. Mur.

Throat, dryness, with rough fauces (back throat), Kali. Mur.

Throat, dryness, without thirst, Nat. Sulph.

Throat, dry, as if from husks of grain, Kali. Mur.

Throat, dry, painful, with chronic catarrh, Silica.

Throat, diphtheretic sore, Nat. Phos.

Throat, diphtheretic sore on soft palate, much swelling, Calc. Sulph., Kali. Mur.

Throat, fauces (back throat), pain in on swallowing, Calc. Phos.

Throat, fauces, redness of, Kali. Mur., Ferr. Phos.

Throat, fauces, secondary syphilis, affecting, Kali. Mur.

Throat, tough slime in, Silica.

Throat, glands of, swollen, Silica, Kali. Mur.

Throat, hemming and hawking constantly to clear, Calc. Phos.

Throat, left side of, sore when swallowing, Silica.

Throat, red and swollen, warm drinks do not hurt, Calc. Phos.

Throat, sore, aching in, worse when swallowing, Calc. Phos.

Throat, sore, as if burned on top, while eating, Calc. Sulph.

Throat, sore, contraction on swallowing saliva, worse talking and swallowing solids, Nat. Sulph.

Throat, sore to the touch, Silica.

Throat, sore, tickling cough, worse in bed, Calc. Phos.

Throat, swelling, in front of, beginning on left and extending to right side, Silica.

Throat, swelling in, that cannot be swallowed, yet constant effort to do so, Nat. Mur.

Throat, troubles, with acid stomach, Nat. Phos.

Throat, weakness in, Calc. Phos.

Throat, worse after retiring, Calc. Phos.

Throat, worse from cold drinks, Calc. Fluor., Silica.

Throat, worse from swallowing liquids, Nat. Phos.

Throat, worse from swallowing solids, Nat. Sulph.

Throat, worse from talking, Nat. Sulph.

Throat, worse from 3 to 4 P. M., Calc. Phos.

Throat, worse in bed, Calc. Phos., Calc. Fluor.

Throat, worse when swallowing, Calc. Phos., Kali. Mur., Nat. Phos., Nat. Mur.

Throat, worse when walking, Nat. Sulph.

Tonsils, chronic swelling of, Calc. Phos.

Tonsils, diphtheretic membrane, on right, Ferr. Phos.

Tonsils, diphtheretic, white patches on, Kali. Mur.

Tonsils, large and sore, especially the left, Kali. Phos.

Tonsils, swollen, with white or grayish-white covering, Kali. Mur.

Tonsils, swollen, swallowing distorts face, Silica.

Tonsils, tight-like exudation on, Ferr. Phos.

Tonsils, ulcers on, tearing pains down throat, Nat. Sulph.

Windpipe, rough, soreness in, and in bronchi, Silica.

Windpipe, sore when coughing, larynx also, Nat. Mur.

CHEST AND LUNGS.

Chest, acute dropsy of lungs, spasmodic cough, face pale, Nat. Sulph., Nat. Mur.

Bleeding of lungs, Ferr. Phos.

Catarrhal consumption of right lung, crackling respiration, pale, emaciated, feverish ; cough, with greenish expectoration, Kali. Mur.

Chest, sore and painful, cavities in lungs, Silica ; from coughing, Mag. Phos.

Chest, worse on motion, Ferr. Phos., Silica.

Chest, worse when coughing, Ferr. Phos.

Cold in lungs, thick, white or yellow expectoration, Kali. Mur.

Consumption, profuse sweat in, cold extremities, Calc. Phos.

Oppression of chest, worse in damp weather, Nat. Sulph.

Oppression of chest, with rush of blood, Ferr. Phos.

Phlegm, rattling in chest, Calc. Phos.

Pleurisy, first stage, Ferr. Phos.

Pleurisy, second stage, Kali. Mur.

Pleurisy, third stage, Nat. Mur.

Pneumonia, chronic, Kali. Sulph.

Pneumonia, bronco., after seeming recovery, but coughs and rattles, Kali. Sulph

Pneumonia, neglected, suppuration, Silica.

Rattling, in chest, when following an acute attack of inflammation, Kali. Sulph.

NOSE.

Difficulty, of breathing or talking through, Nat. Mur.

Dryness and stoppage, after suppressed foot-sweat, Silica.

Foul discharge from bone coverings or sub-mucous connective tissue, Silica.

Foul discharge from syphilitic affections, Nat. Sulph.
Fullness, at root of nose, Nat. Phos.
Interior of, dry, covered with crusts, Silica.
Nostrils, stopped, Kali. Phos., Kali. Mur.
Nose, offensive odor from, in morning, Nat. Phos.
Nose, obstructed nose, sneezes from slight exposure to air, Kali. Phos.
Nose, obstructed in morning, fluent coryza during day, Silica.
Nose, picks at, Nat. Phos.
Nose, red on tip, Silica.
Sneezing, occasionally, with constant desire to do so, Kali. Phos.
Sneezing, spasms of, in morning, Nat. Mur., Silica.
Sneezing, violently, Kali. Phos.
Stoppage, of nose, Nat. Mur., Nat. Sulph.
Sore, internally, Nat. Mur., Silica.
Swollen, red, sore, worse from blowing nose, Nat. Mur.
Take cold in nose easily, Ferr. Phos., Calc. Phos.

Section 8.—Sensations.

BRAIN.—EARS.—EYES.—HEAD.—NERVES.—PAIN.—TASTE.
SENSATIONS IN GENERAL.

BRAIN.

Brain, affections of, with bad-smelling diarrhea, Kali. Phos.
Brain, anæmic, Kali. Phos.
Brain, congestion of, Ferr. Phos.
Brain, concussion of, Kali. Phos., Ferr. Phos.
Brain, crown, pressure on, as if great weight, when going into dark, Silica.
Brain, disease of, with convulsive symptoms, Mag. Phos.

Brain, diseases, paralytic, Silica.
Brain, excess of blood in, Calc. Phos.
Brain-fag, from overwork, Kali. Phos.
Brain-fag, from mental strain, Kali. Phos.
Brain, muddled, thick, Silica.
Brain, fever, Ferr. Phos.
Brain, gnawing pain at base of, or as if in a vice, Nat. Sulph.
Brain, irritation of, after injuries, Nat. Sulph.
Brain, rush of blood to, delirium, Ferr. Phos.
Brain, sharp pain between eyes and back of head, worse at night, Kali. Phos.
Brain, softening of, early stage, Kali Phos.
Brain, softening of, from inflammations, alternate Kali. Phos. with Ferr. Phos.
Brain, softening of, water on, alternate Kali. Phos. with Calc. Phos.
Brain, to prevent dropsy of, Calc. Phos.
Brain, violent pains at base of, Kali. Sulph.
Brain, violent pains at base of, with bilious symptoms, Nat. Sulph.
Brain, water on, Kali. Phos., Nat. Sulph.

EARS.

Child, bores fingers into, or puts hands behind, Silica.
Deafness, from catarrh and swelling of middle ear and canal leading from soft palate to internal ear, Kali. Mur., Silica.
Deafness, from swelling of internal ear, Kali. Mur., Silica.
Deafness, from swelling of external ear, Kali. Sulph., Kali. Mur.

Deafness, from weakness of auditory nerve fibers, Mag. Phos., Kali. Phos.

Deafness, from weakness or exhaustion of auditory nerve, Kali. Phos.

Deafness, with cracking noise when blowing nose, white-coated tongue, Kali. Mur.

Deafness, with evening aggravations, Kali. Sulph.

Deafness, with exhaustion of nervous system, Kali. Phos.

Deafness, with paralysis in ear, Silica.

Deafness, with swelling of glands, Kali. Mur.

Deafness, with thick, yellow discharge, Calc. Sulph.

Deafness, without noise in ear, disappearing when blowing nose or coughing, Silica.

Deafness, relieved by electricity, Silica.

Deafness, from thickening of drum membrane, Kali. Mur.

Ears, sore, swollen, itching and hot, Calc. Phos.

Ears, worse at night, changing weather, or sitting long, Silica.

Ears, worse from washing or changing linen, Silica.

Ear-wax, dark, from right ear in morning, Calc. Sulph.

Ear-wax, secretion of increased, Silica.

Hearing, difficult, Calc. Phos., Nat. Mur., Silica.

Hearing, difficult, after fainting, Silica.

Hearing, difficult, after over-exertion, Silica.

Hearing, difficult, after over-exertion, with heaviness in head, Silica.

Hearing, difficult, especially of human voice, and during full moon, Silica.

Hearing, difficult, from swelling of tympanic cavity, Silica, Kali. Mur.

Hearing, difficult, of nervous origin, Silica, Kali. Phos.

Hearing, difficult, with noises in head, Kali. Phos.

Hearing, difficult, caused by roaring in head; Silica.

Hearing, supersensitive, cannot bear noises, Kali. Phos.

One ear red and hot, frequently itches, with stomach derangements and acid conditions, Nat. Phos.

Outer ear, sore and scaly, Nat. Phos.

Outer ear, sore, with creamy discharge, Nat. Phos.

Oversensitiveness of ears, Kali. Phos., Silica.

Soreness in and around ears, Calc. Phos.

EYES.

Angles of, red and sore from acrid tears, Nat. Mur.

Aversion of, to light. Calc. Phos.

Blackness, sudden, things turn dark, Nat. Mur.

Black spots before, Silica.

Black spots or streaks of light around objects, Nat. Mur.

Blindness, during day, with sudden appearance of boils, Silica.

Blindness, occasional, with twitching of lids, Calc. Sulph., Mag. Phos.

Blindness, sudden, momentary, Silica.

Blindness, from partial decay of optic nerve, Kali. Phos.

Blood-shot eyes, Ferr. Phs.

Blood-shot eyes, with burning tears, Nat. Phos.

Blurred vision, after straining eyes, Calc. Fluor.

Candle light hurts eyes, Calc. Phos.

Catarrhal contraction of tear duct, Nat. Mur., Kali. Mur.

Child buries head in pillow (ulceration of cornea), Nat. Mur.

Colors before eyes, Mag. Phos.

Conjunctiva, swollen, protruding, muco-purulent discharge, Nat. Mur.

Conjunctiva, yellow, Nat. Sulph.

Congestion of eyes, Kali. Mur., Ferr. Phos.

Contracted pupils, Mag. Phos., Nat. Mur.

Cracks in angles of lids, Nat. Mur.

Daylight dazzles, Silica.

Double sight (diplopia), objects seen double, Mag. Phos., Calc. Phos.

Drooping of eye-lids, Kali. Phos., Mag. Phos.

Dryness and burning in eyes, worse afternoon and evening, Nat. Sulph.

Dryness of left eye-ball, soreness, Nat. Phos.

Dull sight, from weak optic nerve, Mag. Phos.

Eruption of small vesicles, causing scalding tears, Nat. Mur.

Excited, staring appearance of eyes, Kali. Phos.

Eye-balls, dryness of left, sore, as if bruised, Nat. Phos.

Eye-balls, distorted, as from pressure, Calc. Phos.

Eye-balls, protrude, Kali. Mur., Calc. Sulph.

Eye-balls, sore, when reading, worse from gaslight, Nat. Phos.

Eye-balls, sore, worse from pressure, Ferr. Phos., Kali. Phos.

Eye-balls, yellow, from bad liver, Nat. Sulph.

Eyelids, catarrhal affections of, lids red, burn while reading, Nat. Mur.

Eyelids, corners and borders raw and ulcerated, Nat. Mur.

Eyelids, edges of, burn, Kali. Sulph.

Eyelids, edges of, scabby, Kali. Mur.

Eyelids, glutinous substance collects in corners, Nat. Mur.

Eyelids, granulations on, Ferr. Phos., Kali. Mur.

Eyelids, heavy motion of, Kali. Phos.

Eyelids, indurations around, Silica.

Eyelids, neuralgia of, Mag. Phos., Nat. Mur., Silica.

Eyelids, painless swelling of, Silica, Kali. Mur.

Eyelids, smarting and soreness of, Silica.

Eyelids, sore, red, look like raw beef, Ferr. Phos., Nat. Mur.

Eyelids, specks of matter on, yellow, mattery scabs, Kali. Mur.

Eyelids, stick together in morning, Nat. Mur., Nat. Phos.

Eyelids, swollen, excessive tears, corners cracked, Nat. Mur.

Eyelids, turned in, after caustic treatment of granular lids, Silica.

Eyes, give out when reading or writing, Nat. Mur.

Eyes, hollow, sunken, Kali. Phos.

Eyes, red and bleared, with colic, Calc. Sulph.

Eyes, ulcereted and raw, Nat. Mur.

Flickering before, misty, Silica, Calc. Fluor.

Flickering, in left, at 5 A. M., Nat. Phos.

Granular lids, chronic, Nat. Mur.

Granulations, blister like, blinding tears, Nat. Mur.

Granulations, blister like, burning tears, Nat. Sulph.

Halo around gaslight, Nat. Phos.

Hypopyon (an accumulation in the anterior of the eye), Calc. Sulph.

Haziness of sight, Calc. Phos.

Intolerance of light, Ferr. Phos., Calc. Phos.

Iris, discolored, Nat. Mur.

Left cornea hazy, averse to light, Calc. Phos.

Left eye, soreness in, in evening, Calc. Sulph.

Letters and stitches run together, Nat. Mur.

Letters change into small points, Calc. Phos.

Letters look pale, Silica.

Lightning-like flashes, vision obscured, Silica.

Luminous appearance on coughing or sneezing, Kali. Mur.

Objects appear perpendicular, Nat. Mur.

Objects swim, or become confused, Nat. Mur.

Optical defects, cause vertigo, Mag. Phos.

Pupils, contracted, Mag. Phos.

Pupils, dilated, excited, staring appearance, Kali. Phos.

Pupils, dilate during disease, Kali. Mur.

Redness of eyes, in evening, Kali. Mur., Nat. Mur.

Redness of whites, with pressing pain or excessive tears, Nat. Mur., Ferr. Phos.

Right eye, persistent speck before, Silica.

Sees only half an object, Calc. Sulph., Nat. Mur.

Sensitive to light, Calc. Phos., Mag. Phos., Nat. Mur., Nat. Sulph., Silica.

Sight, illusion of, Mag. Phos.

Sight, momentary loss of, with uterine troubles, pregnancy, Silica.

Sight, obscured, worse when stooping, walking, reading or writing, Nat. Mur.

Sight, weak, from exhausted optic nerve, Kali. Phos.

Sight, weak, after diphtheria, Kali. Phos., Silica.

Sight, weak, from use of stimulants, Silica.

Slight fluttering before eyes, Silica.

Spots or scars on cornea, Silica, Calc. Fluor.

Streaks of light around objects, Nat. Mur.

Stricture of tear duct, Nat. Mur.

Symptoms, alternate from one eye to the other, Silica.

Tears, excessive, from weakness, in open air, Nat. Mur.

Thick, rough, warty cornea, Silica.

Troubles, reflex, from uterine irritation, Nat. Mur.

Unsteadiness of sight, Nat. Mur.

Veil, before eyes, Calc. Phos.

Veil, before eyes, at 10 A. M., Nat. Mur.

Vision, dim, as if looking through a veil, Nat. Phos.

Vision, dim, as if looking through gauze or feathers, Nat. Mur.

Vision, dim, after suppressed foot-sweat, Silica.

Vision, indistinct, misty, Silica., Calc. Phos.

Vision, weak, from nervous losses, Nat. Mur.

Vision, weak, in nervous, sensitive persons, Silica, Kali. Phos.

Vision, spasmodic, of sparks or rainbow colors, Mag. Phos.

Weak and watering eyes, Nat. Mur.

HEAD.

Head, chronic effects of injuries, Nat. Mur.

Head, debilitated conditions, Kali. Phos.

Head, falls forward in spinal disease, Silica.

Head, troubles less when wrapped warmly, worse in winter, Silica.

Head, inability to hold up, Calc. Phos.

Head, jerks to right side, Nat. Sulph.

Head, jerking in chorea, Nat. Mur.

Head, nods forward from weakness, Nat. Mur.

Head, rolls from side to side, Silica.

Head, stuffy cold in, white, grayish tongue, Kali. Mur.

Head, top cold and sensitive, Nat. Mur.

Head, top sensitive to cold air, noise, or any jar, Ferr. Phos.

Head, soreness in, Ferr. Phos.

Head, too large, body emaciated, face pale, abdomen hot and bloated, Silica.

Head, weariness in, Nat. Mur.

NERVES.

Acute, weakening diseases, Calc. Phos.

All ailments, with want of nerve power, nervous prostration, exhaustion, nervous rigors, Kali. Phos.

Anxiety, nervous dread without special cause, gloomy moods, fancies, dark forebodings, Kali. Phos.

Assimilation, imperfect in over-sensitive persons, constipation, neuralgia, melancholy, Silica.

Better, from continued gentle motion, Kali. Phos.

Body, restlessnessness of when sitting long, Silica.

Body, trembling, Nat. Mur., Nat. Sulph.

Body, bruised pain over, Silica.

Chattering of teeth, nervous, not from cold, Kali. Phos.

Chorea (St. Vitus dance), involuntary movements and contortions of limbs, Mag. Phos.

Collapse, livid, bluish countenance, and low pulse, Kali. Phos.

Convulsions, at full moon, Silica.

Convulsions, followed by delirium, Kali. Mur.

Convulsions, with fever, Ferr. Phos.

Convulsions, with stiff limbs, fingers clenched, Mag. Phos.

Cramps, Mag. Phos.

Creeping numbness, Calc. Phos.

Creeping paralysis, wasting, unconscious to touch, Kali. Phos.

Debility and sleepiness in thunder storm, Silica.

Debility, from loss of fluids, after masturbation, Nat. Mur.

Debility, hysterical, worse in morning, Nat. Mur.

Debility, of children with no organic trouble, Ferr. Phos.

Debility, with great weakness, Silica.

Debility, with incontinence of urine, Calc. Phos.

Debility, with nervousness and irritability, Kali. Phos.

Delirium tremens, fear, sleeplessness, restlessness, rambling talk, visionary images, Kali. Phos., Nat. Mur.

Depression and lassitude, Kali. Phos.

Despondent, dwells upon grievances, Kali. Phos.

Desire to stretch, Calc. Phos.

Dread of noise or light, Kali Phos.

Drops things from nervous weakness, Nat. Mur.

Epilepsy, Calc. Phos., Ferr. Phos., Kali. Phos., Mag. Phos., Nat. Mur., Nat. Sulph., Silica.

Epilepsy, after suppressed eruptions, Kali. Mur.

Epilepsy, at night, or new moon, preceded by coldness of left side, Silica.

Epilepsy, from slight provocation, Silica, Mag. Phos., Calc. Phos., Kali. Mur.

Epilepsy, from local irritation of nerves, Mag. Phos.

Epilepsy, in general, Mag. Phos.

Epilepsy, in scrofulous or young persons growing too fast, Calc. Phos.

Epilepsy, with or after eczema, Kali. Mur.

Epilepsy, from vicious habits, Mag. Phos., and restraint.

Epilepsy, when an over-excited, not depressed, condition of the nerves exists, Mag. Phos.

Epilepsy, with bulging of eye-balls, Kali. Mur.

Epilepsy, with congestion to head, Ferr. Phos.

Epilepsy, with pallor, sunken countenance, coldness and palpitation after fit, Kali. Phos.

Epilepsy, white, coated tongue, Kali. Mur.

Epilepsy, fits of, falling sickness, from abnormal condition of nerve cells, with cold limbs, great pallor, and shrunken face, Kali. Phos.

Epilepsy, with clenched fists or teeth, stiff limbs, Mag. Phos., sometimes Calc. Phos. also.

Exhaustion, after dreams, Calc. Sulph.

Exhaustion, with colic, Nat. Sulph.

Exhaustion, with unusual irritability, Silica.

Faintness, in nervous people, Kali. Phos.

Faintness, lassitude and palpitation, Kali. Phos.

Fatigue, all day, Calc. Fluor.

Fatigued, easily, lassitude after rising, Nat. Mur.

Feeling, as of a ball rising in throat, Kali. Phos.

Feels pain keenly, Kali. Phos.

Feels prostrated, as if beaten all over, Silica.

Feet and hands, twitch during sleep, Nat. Sulph.

Fidgety, restless, starts at least noise, Kali. Phos., Silica.

Fits, where the lime salts are at fault, Calc. Phos.

Fits, from fright, pallid or livid countenance, Kali. Phos.

Fits, in the strumous and scrofulous, Calc. Phos.

Great debility, inclined to weep, Nat. Mur.

Great weakness in morning, Silica.

Head, involuntary shaking of, Mag. Phos.

Heart, palpitation or trembling of, Nat. Phos.

Hysteria, Nat. Mur., Kali. Phos.

Hysteria, from sudden or intense emotion, hysterical fits of laughing and crying, Kali. Phos.

Hysterical spasms, developing into severe convulsions, Nat. Mur.

Impatient, irritable, Kali. Phos.

Internal restlessness and excitement, Silica.

Jerking of right side and head, Nat. Mur.

Languid, weak, no pluck, Calc. Phos.

Languid, weak, with malarial symptoms, Nat. Sulph.

Lassitude, Nat. Sulph.

Makes mountains out of mole hills, Kali. Phos.

Nervousness, Kali. Phos

Nervous, from sudden or intense emotions, or from smothering passion, Kali. Phos.

Nervous debility, Nat. Phos.

Nervous debility, emaciation, faint when lying on side, Silica.

Nervous, in thunder storm, Nat. Phos.

Nervous-sensitiveness, Kali. Phos.

Numbness, after unpleasant news, Calc. Phos.

Numb feeling, in affected part, Nat Mur.

Oppression and weakness from head to stomach, Calc. Sulph.

Overstrained easily by lifting, Silica.

Palsy, Mag Phos.

Paralysis, from anger or emotion, Nat Mur., Kali. Phos.

Paralysis, from sexual excesses or other nervous exhaustion, Nat. Mur., Kali. Phos.

Paralysis, of bladder, Silica.

Paralysis, of face commencing with faceache, tender to touch or pressure, Kali. Mur.

Paralysis, of hands, Silica.

Paralysis, of retina, Calc. Phos., Kali. Phos.

Paralysis, rheumatic. acute cases of, Ferr. Phos.

Paralytic states, Kali. Phos.

Prostrated, Silica.

Prostration, great, during summer complaint, Ferr. Phos.

Restlessness, after sitting long, Silica.

Restlessness, with chilliness, moves limbs constantly, Nat. Mur.

Restlessness, with pains in liver, tired, backache, Calc. Fluor.

Sciatica, affection of sciatic nerve, Kali. Phos.

Sciatica, chief remedies : Kali. Phos., Mag. Phos., Nat. Sulph.

Sciatica, dragging pain, torpor, stiffness. Kali. Phos.

Sciatica, great restlessness and pain, Kali. Phos.

Sciatica, gentle motion gives relief, continued exercise makes worse, Kali. Phos.

Sciatica, lack of moving power, Kali. Phos.

Sciatica, nervous exhaustion, Kali Phos.

Sciatica, neuralgic or rheumatic affections of sciatic nerve, Kali. Phos., Mag. Phos

Sciatica, no relief in any position, Nat. Sulph.

Sciatica, with symptoms of gout, alternate Nat. Sulph. and Kali. Phos.

Sciatica, worse when rising from a sitting position, Nat. Sulph.

Shaking and trembling of hands, limbs or head (palsy), Mag. Phos.

Shaking, spasmodic trembling, from want of nervous control, Mag. Phos.

Shyness, excessive blushing; from undue sensitiveness of nerves, Kali. Phos.

Spasms, chronic or hysterical, Nat. Mur.

Spasms, during full moon, Nat. Mur., Silica.

Spasms, followed by sensitiveness, especially to noise, suspicious, fearful, Mag. Phos., Kali. Phos.

Spasms, from water on brain, Nat. Mur., Nat. Sulph.

Spasms, in feverish diseases, Nat. Mur.

Spasms, like an electric shock, Calc. Phos.

Spasms, occurring at night, Silica, Mag. Phos., Calc. Phos.

Spasms, with contraction of fingers, staring eyes, spasmodic cough, Mag. Phos.

Spasmodic, convulsive sobbing, Mag. Phos.

Spasmodic muscular contractions, Mag. Phos.

Spinal debility, from exhausting diseases, Kali. Phos.

Starting, by touch, or at sudden noise, Kali. Phos., Silica.

Starting, in sleep, Calc. Phos.

Talking in sleep, and restless nights, Nat. Mur.

Tired, weary and exhausted, Calc. Phos., Mag. Phos., Kali. Phos.

Tired, weary, especially in knees, Nat. Sulph.

Tired, weary, with biliousness, Nat. Sulph.

Tired, with gone feeling at stomach, trembling, Nat. Phos.

Trembling in nerves, at night, Kali. Phos., Nat. Mur.

Unrefreshed in morning, Calc. Fluor., Nat. Mur., Silica.

Visions, in sleep, Nat. Mur.

Whining and fretful disposition, Kali. Phos.

Writer's cramp, Mag. Phos.

Yawning and stretching, Nat. Mur.

Yawning, unnatural, excessive, hysterical, Kali. Phos.

PAIN.

Abdomen, aching, burning pains in groins, Calc. Phos.

Abdomen, bearing-down pains, worse on left side near groin, Kali. Phos.

Abdomen, colicky pains in right groin, extending over whole abdomen, Nat. Sulph.

Abdomen, contractive pain in, before stool, Nat. Mur., Nat. Sulph.

Abdomen, contractive pain in, extending to chest, tight breath, followed by diarrhea, Nat. Sulph.

Abdomen, cutting and griping, with rumbling in, Nat. Mur.

Abdomen, cutting pains in, Nat. Sulph., Mag. Phos., Ferr. Phos.

Abdomen, cramps in, pains around and above navel' Mag. Phos.

Abdomen, dull, heavy pain from abdomen to back, Nat. Sulph.

Abdomen, pains in, better from warmth or friction, Mag. Phos., Silica.

Abdomen, pain in, with melancholy, Nat. Mur.

Abdomen, pain in, with soft stools, Kali. Mur.

Abdomen, pinching pain in right side of, Nat. Mur.

Abdomen, pressive pain in, Silica.

Abdomen, shooting, contracting pains, Mag. Phos.

Acute or chronic pains, Ferr. Phos.

Ankles, cramp-like pains in, Calc. Phos.

Ankles, pain, as if sprained, Nat. Mur.

Ankles, pain in, and in shins, knees, hollow and ball of foot, Nat. Phos.

Ankles, pain, rending, tearing, shooting in, Calc. Phos.

Ankles, pain, spasmodic, Mag. Phos.

Anus, contracting, lancinating pains in during stool, Nat. Mur.

Anus, crampy pains from, into rectum and testicles; Silica.

Anus, pains during stool, as if constricted, Silica.

Arm, aching, bruised, sore pain in, Calc. Phos.

Arm, dull pains in, worse from changing weather, Calc. Phos.

Arm, go to sleep when resting on, pricking in, Silica.

Arm, pain in, better from warmth, Silica.

Arm, shooting and tearing from shoulder down, Calc. Phos.

Back, pains in, Nat. Mur.

Bladder, cutting pain in, and in urethra, Kali. Phos., Nat. Mur.

Bladder, cutting and burning, after urinating, Nat. Mur., Calc. Phos.

Bladder, cutting pains while urinating, Silica.

Bladder, pain and pressure in after urinating, Calc. Phos.

Bladder, pain violent, with weak stream of water, Calc. Phos.

Bladder, shooting in mouth of, Calc. Phos.

Bladder, sore, aching, worse after urinating. Calc. Phos.

Bladder, stitches in, and in urethra, Kali. Phos.

Bones, long, pain in, Nat. Phos.

Bones, shin, pain in, Calc. Phos.

Bowels, bruised, pain in, Nat. Sulph.

Bowels, neuralgia of, Mag. Phos.

Bowels, pains in, restless sleep, Nat. Phos.

Bowels, pinching in, with pain in forehead, rumbling, shifting pain, followed by diarrhea, Nat. Sulph.

Chest, ache in lower, extending upwards, Calc. Phos.

Chest, ache in left upper, through to shoulder blade, Calc. Phos. ; worse from motion and pressure, Kali. Phos.

Chest, ache, with soreness to touch, Calc. Phos., Kali. Phos.

Chest, cutting, crampy pain from left chest through to shoulder, Nat. Mur.

Chest, excruciating, deep-seated pain in, Silica.

Chest, pain in, with headache, Calc. Sulph

Chest, pain in lower left, worse by coughing, dry tongue, frequent intermittent pulse, loss of appetite, weakness, Calc. Fluor.

Chest, painful stinging in, and in sides, Kali. Phos.

Chest, sharp, cutting, transitory pains, low in right chest, Kali. Phos.

Chest, sharp pain in middle right chest, later in left, in—

termittent, takes away breath, worse with deep breathing, and in day, Calc. Phos.

Chest, sharp pain in end of breast bone during day, Calc. Phos.

Chest, shooting from breast bone around to back, Silica.

Chest, sticking in on breathing, or through to back, Silica.

Chest, stitches in chest and side on breathing, with cough, Nat. Mur.

Chest, stitches in breast bone, or under left ribs, Nat. Mur.

Chest, stitches in left side, when breathing, Calc. Phos., Kali. Phos.

Chest, tensive pain across, lasting several hours, Silica.

Chest, weakness in, pains, stitches, can hardly speak, Silica.

Ear, aching, itching in right opening, Nat. Phos.

Ear, itching and prickling, Silica.

Ear, itching, pressing, mostly in left, Silica.

Ear, itching, rending, pressing. in and around, Calc. Phos.

Ear, beating and throbbing in, red from congestion, Nat. Mur.

Ear, boring pains, bores fingers into, Silica.

Ear, cutting pain under, Kali. Sulph.

Ear, drawing, shooting pains in, worse at night, change in weather, motion, etc., Silica.

Ear, drawing, stitching pains from ear to neck and shoulder, Nat. Mur.

Ear, inflammatory pains in, Ferr. Phos.

Ear, neuralgic pains in and around, Mag. Phos.

Ear, nervous, spasmodic, Mag. Phos.

Earache, aggravated by cold, relieved by heat, Mag. Phos.

Earache, aggravated by damp weather, Nat. Sulph.

Earache, as if something forcing its way out, Nat. Sulph.

Earache, beating, throbbing pain, Ferr. Phos.

Earache, inflammatory, from cold, with burning or throbbing pains, Ferr. Phos.

Earache, lightning-like pain, Nat. Sulph.

Earache, outer aching, with heat or coldness, Calc. Phos.

Earache, pain deep-seated, stinging, itching, worse lying down, Kali. Phos.

Earache, pain in bones around ears, shooting upwards, Calc. Phos.

Earache, pain in disturbs sleep, Silica.

Earache, piercing in right, inward, Nat. Sulph.

Earache, sharp, lightning-like stitches, worse changing from cold to warm air, and in damp weather, Nat. Sulph.

Earache, sharp pain in left, and down cheek, Kali. Phos.

Earache, sharp pain under, cutting and stitching, Kali. Sulph.

Earache, stitching pain in, Ferr. Phos.

Earache, tearing, shooting, jerking pain, alternating with rheumatic troubles, Calc. Phos.

Earache, with cracking noises in ears while swallowing, Kali. Mur.

Earache, with discharge of watery or yellow matter, Kali. Sulph.

Earache, with swelling of glands or throat, Kali. Mur.

Earache, with white, furred tongue, Kali. Mur.

Elbows, shooting through, Calc. Phos.

Eyes, aching in back head, corresponding to eye affected, Silica.

Eyes, ache, after steady use, Calc. Fluor

Eyes, acute pain, worse from motion or use, Ferr. Phos.

Eyes, cutting, stitching, burning pain, Nat. Phos.

Eyes, dull, continual over right, Calc. Sulph.

Eyes, neuralgia over, darting pains on exposure to light, or before a storm, Silica.

Eyes, neuralgia of, periodic, with flow of tears and red conjunctiva, Nat. Mur.

Eyes, neuralgic pains in, Mag. Phos.; if that fails, Calc. Phos.

Eyes, neuralgic pains in, with excessive tears, Nat. Mur.

Eyes, pain, paroxysms of tearing, shooting, throbbing, Silica, Mag. Phos.

Eyes, pain, pressive over, Silica.

Eyes, pain severe, great redness, no mucous or matter, Ferr. Phos.

Eyes, pain severe through, worse in sunlight, Kali. Phos.

Eyes, pains in and above, begin and end with the sun, Nat. Mur.

Eyes, pains over, Calc. Sulph., Mag. Phos., Nat. Mur.

Eyes, painful, as if too dry and full of sand, Silica.

Eyes, piercing, stinging pain in, Silica.

Eyes, severe pain from, into head, better from warmth, Silica.

Eyes, sharp, piercing pain above when looking down, ulceration of cornea, Nat. Mur.

Eyes, stitches in temples when looking at the light, Nat. Mur.

Eyes, stitches over, Nat. Mur.

Eyes, stitches through, and in cheek bones, Silica.

Eyeballs, ache, as if beaten, Calc. Phos., Kali. Phos.

Eyeballs, ache, when looking intently, Nat. Mur.

Eyeballs, dull, pressive pain in, lids raised with difficulty, Nat. Mur.

Eyeballs, pain in, aggravated by movement, and relieved by cold water, Ferr. Phos.

Eyeballs, pain in, relieved by resting, Calc. Fluor.

Face, grinding pain in, Mag. Phos., Calc. Phos.

Face, neuralgia of, Kali. Phos., Nat. Mur., Mag. Phos., Nat. Phos., Silica.

Face, neuralgia of, accompanied by earache, Mag. Phos.

Face, neuralgia of, accompanied by flow of tears, Nat. Mur.

Face, neuralgia of, accompanied by shifting pains, Mag. Phos., Kali. Sulph.

Face, neuralgia of, accompanied by shooting, spasmodic pains, Mag. Phos.

Face, neuralgia of, from exposure to wind, Mag. Phos.

Face, neuralgia of, from exhaustion of nervous system, Kali. Phos.

Face, neuralgia of, regularly at 7 A. M , increased until noon, then decreases, Nat. Mur.

. Face, neuralgia of, right side, flying pains, Mag. Phos.

Face, neuralgia of, right side, relieved by cold applications, Kali. Phos.

Face, neuralgia of, shooting, stitching pains, Nat. Phos.

Face, neuralgia of, with great weakness after, Kali. Phos.

Face, neuralgia of, worse from cold or touch, Mag. Phos.

Face, neuralgia of, worse in heated room, or evening, Kali. Sulph.

Face, pain in. especially under jawbone, Calc. Phos.

Face, pain in right upper jaw, Calc. Sulph.

Face, pains darting, shooting, crampy, right side swollen, Mag. Phos.

Face, tearing pain in, Mag. Phos., Calc. Sulph.

Face-ache, accompanied by constipation, Nat. Mur.

Face-ache, accompanied by flow of tears, Nat. Mur.

Face-ache, accompanied by rheumatic pains, Mag. Phos.

Face-ache, accompanied by small lumps on face, Silica.

Face-ache, accompanied by vomiting of clear mucous, Nat. Mur.

Face-ache, from swelling of cheek, Kali. Mur.

Face-ache, neuralgic or rheumatic, worse at night, Calc. Phos.

Face-ache, worse in warm room, or evening, better in cool, open air, Kali. Sulph.

Feet, drawing pains in soles of, Kali. Phos.

Feet, great pain, shooting up inside of leg, Ferr. Phos.

Feet, pains through, Silica.

Feet, pains in hollow and ball, Nat. Phos.

Feet, painful spasm in while walking, Silica.

Feet, piercing in soles and heels, ulcerative pains, Nat. Sulph.

Feet, severe shooting in and around ankle, Ferr. Phos.

Feet, shooting in soles, and balls of toes, Calc. Phos.

Feet, stinging in, Calc. Phos.

Feet, stitches in soles, severe, Silica.

Feet, walking painful, sore from instep through to sole, Silica.

Fingers, sticking pains, as if asleep, Silica.

Gland, under ear, aching in, Calc. Phos.

Gland, under jaw, painful to touch, not swollen, Silica.

Hands, cramp-like pain and lameness, Silica.

Hands, crampy pains when witring, trembling, Silica.

Heart, cutting, shooting in region of, interrupts breathing, Calc. Phos.

Heart, pain from front of, down to thigh, Calc. Sulph.

Heart, sharp pains in, Calc. Phos.

Heart, sharp, shooting, darting pains, Mag. Phos.

Heart, stitches in after reading aloud, Nat. Mur.

Head, bending down causes pain, Nat. Mur.

Head, brain, gnawing pain at base of, or as if in a vice, Nat. Sulph.

Head, brain, irritation of, after injuries, Nat. Sulph.

Head, brain, sharp pain through base, between eyes and back head, worse at night, Kali. Phos.

Head, brain, violent pains at base of, Kali. Sulph.

Head, brain, violent pains at base of, with bilious symptoms, Nat Sulph.

Head, dull, heavy pain on top of, during profuse menses, Ferr. Phos.

Head, flashes of pain through, also eyes and neck, Mag. Phos.

Head, forehead, hammering in, and in temples, worse in right, fears apoplexy, Ferr. Phos.

Head, forehead, tearing in, stitching, Silica.

Head, forehead, tension in, throbbing and pounding, Silica.

Head, left temple, aching in, Kali. Mur.

Head, left temple, severe, sharp, transitory pains in, Kali. Phos.

Head, movement of causes pain, Nat. Sulph.

Head, moves forward without pain, backward or sideways with pain, Nat. Sulph.

Head, neck, sharp pain in nape of, Mag. Phos.

Head, neuralgia in, Calc. Phos., Ferr. Phos., Mag. Phos.

Head, neuralgia of left side, worse by motion, and in open air, Kali. Phos.

Head, neuralgia of whole, eyes, teeth and ears, worse at night, Silica.

Head, nose-bleed relieves pain in, Ferr. Phos.

Head, pains in, and in face, with hawking of white mucous, Kali. Mur.

Head, pains in, from hunger, Silica.

Head, pains in, aggravated by cold, Mag. Phos.

Head, pains in, better by gentle excitement or motion, Kali. Phos.

Head, pains in, better by heat, Mag. Phos.

Head, right temple, boring in, preceded by burning at pit of stomach, lassitude, at night or morning, Nat. Sulph.

Head, sharp pain from back to front on stooping, Ferr. Phos.

Head, shooting, stinging, shifting, intermittent, or spasmodic pains, Mag. Phos.

Head, stitching in, Nat. Mur.

Head, stinging, pressing, throbbing pains, headache or neuralgia of face, aggravated by motion, Ferr. Phos.

Head, temples, fluttering in and aching in back head, Silica.

Head, temple, hammering in, worse on right side, Ferr. Phos.

Head, temples, sharp pain through, Kali. Phos.

Head, temples, stitches in, Silica.

Head, tearing from back over whole head, bursting, throbbing, Silica.

Head, throbbing and heat in back head, Nat. Mur.

Headache, above eyes, can hardly open them, Silica.

Headache, across eyes, dull, fullness, and in both temples, Kali. Phos.

Headache, aching, drawing pains around back head, Calc Phos.

Headache, after rich food, Nat. Mur.

Headache, after sneezing, Nat. Mur.

Headache, after sour milk, Nat. Phos.

Headache, as if brain and eyes were forced forward, Silica.

Headache, as if would burst, Nat. Mur.

Headache, as if rope around head were tighter and tighter, feel as if stepping on air, Nat. Mur.

Headache, as if nail was driven in left side of head, Nat. Mur.

Headache, as if brain fell to left side on stooping, Nat. Sulph.

Headache, as of brain pressing against skull, Calc. Phos.

Headache, back head ache, Kali. Mur., Silica

Headache, back head ache, with great fullness, Ferr. Phos.

Headache, begins with blindness, Nat. Mur.

Headache, begins before and lasts through menses, better from hot applications, lying down, gentle motion, and eating, Kali. Phos.

Headache, better from warmth, Mag. Phos.

Headache, blinding ache, with dull, constant ovarian pain and bearing down, Nat. Mur.

Headache, blind, sick headache, vomiting of undigested food, Ferr. Phos.

Headache, bruising, pressing, stitching pain, worse on movement or by stooping, Ferr. Phos.

Headache, caused by changing weather, Calc. Phos.

Headache, caused by optical defects, Mag. Phos.

Headache, caused or accompanied by biliousness, bitter taste, greenish-gray tongue, Nat. Sulph.

Headache, chronic, from injury to head, Nat. Mur.

Headache, congestive, Ferr. Phos., Silica.

Headache, crown, morning headache, with moist, yellow, creamy coat on back of tongue and roof of mouth, Nat. Phos.

Headache, dull, forgetful, irritable, Mag. Phos.

Headache, dull, with vertigo, flickering before eyes, Nat. Mur.

Headache, dull, almost constant, malarial symptoms, Nat. Mur.

Headache, dull, heavy, with profusion of tears, drowsiness and unrefreshing sleep, Nat. Mur.

Headache, during menses, face red, nausea and vomiting, Nat. Mur.

Headache, epileptic, Ferr. Phos.

Headache, extends into jaws, Kali. Mur.

Headache, frontal, followed and relieved by nose-bleed, Ferr. Phos.

Headache, frontal, or back, with great fullness, Ferr. Phos.

Headache, frontal, pressure, throbbing, dragging, Nat. Mur.

Headache, frontal, worse after dinner, and in evening, Calc. Sulph.

Headache, from brain-fag, of students, Kali. Phos.

Headache, from concussion, eyes feel sunken, pain in chest during menses, Calc. Sulph.

Headache, constipation, torpidity and dryness of intestinal tract, tongue clean, or covered with frothy saliva, Nat. Mur.

Headache, from excessive cold, Ferr. Phos.

Headache, from hunger, Silica.

Headache, from loss of sleep, Kali. Phos.

Headache, from mental work, overstrain of mind, Kali. Phos.

Headache, from nervous prostration, Silica., Kali. Phos.

Headache, from rush of blood to head, cold applications relieve, Ferr. Phos.

Headache, from sun heat, Ferr. Phos.

Headache, followed by vomiting of bile, Nat. Sulph.

Headache, followed by exhaustion, Kali. Phos.

Headache, followed by severe pain in small of back, Silica.

Headache, half headache, sour vomiting, eructations, bloated abdomen, unconscious twitching limbs, Nat. Mur.

Headache, heavy, nose-bleed no relief, Nat. Mur., Nat. Sulph.

Headache, heat relieves and cold makes worse, Mag. Phos.; if not relieved by Mag. Phos., Calc. Phos.

Headache, in forehead, as if from a blow, Nat. Mur.

Headache, in back of head, with weary, exhausted feeling, Kali. Phos.

Headache, in left forehead and head, Calc. Sulph.

Headache, in forehead and eyeballs, lids only raised with pain, Nat. Mur.

Headache, in temples, Nat. Phos.; left temple, Kali. Mur.; sharp, Kali. Phos.

Headache, in evening, with shivering and coldness of body, Silica.

Headache, intense, from emotions or physical exertion, Kali. Phos.

Headache, nervous, excruciating, oversensitiveness to noise, during menses, Kali. Phos.

Headache, with sparks before eyes, Mag. Phos.

Headache, with inability for thought, loss of strength, sleeplessness, Kali. Phos.

Headache, neuralgic, with excruciating, darting, stinging, intermittent or paroxysmal pains, Mag. Phos.

Headache, neuralgic, with humming in the ears, nervousness, Kali. Phos.

Headache, neuralgic, better from warmth, Mag. Phos.

Headache, neuralgic, if not relieved by Mag. Phos., Calc. Phos.

Headache, of nervous subjects, pale, irritable and excitable, Kali. Phos:

Headache, of girls at puberty, Nat. Mur., Calc. Phos.

Headache, of school girls, with diarrhea, Calc. Phos.

Headache, of school girls, during menses, with burning on crown, Nat. Mur.

Headache, on crown of head, Nat. Phos.

Headache, on top, back and forehead, Silica.

Headache, on top and behind ears, neck muscles draw, Calc. Phos.

Headache, on top, with pressure or heat, Nat. Phos.

Headache, one-sided, as if beaten, Silica.

Headache, over forehead, with tearing pains in arms and hands, Calc. Phos.

Headache, over whole head, Calc. Fluor.

Headache, of both sides, as if in a vice, Nat: Mur.

Headache, paralytic, Silica.

Headacne, periodic, throbbing in forehead, at night, with nausea and vomiting, Calc. Sulph.

Headache, pulsating, with congestion, Nat. Sulph.

Headache, pulsating in forehead and top head, chilliness, Silica.

Headache, rheumatic, very severe, Mag. Phos.

Headache, rheumatic, with evening aggravations, Kali. Sulph., Silica.

Headache, rheumatic, worse in warm room, and evening, better in open air, Kali. Sulph.

Headache, rising from neck to top head, Silica.

Headache, severe pain at base of brain and on top, Nat. Sulph.

Headache, sharp, darting over left eye, or in left temple, Kali. Phos.

Headache, sharp, from eyes to back head, better after eating and gentle motion, worse at night, Kali. Phos.

Headache, sick, from sluggish action of liver, Kali. Mur.

Headache, sick, with bitter taste in mouth, Nat. Sulph.

Headache, sick, with biliousness, colicky pains, or bilious diarrhea, Nat. Sulph.

Headache, sick, with vomiting of sour fluids, Nat. Phos.

Headache, sick, with vomiting of undigested food, Nat. Phos., Ferr. Phos.

Headache, sick, with white tongue, vomiting white phlegm, Kali. Mur.

Headache, splitting pain on top, Nat. Sulph.

Headache, stitching, as of knives, in back head, Nat. Mur.

Headache, stitching in the eyes and cheek bones, Silica.

Headache, stops on one side, and worse on the other, Nat. Mur.

Headache, tearing, throbbing, bursting, better from bandaging tightly, Silica.

Headache, throbbing, beating, relieved by cold, Ferr. Phos.

Headache, throbbing, as from little hammers, Nat. Mur.

Headache, with or followed by severe pain in small of back, Silica.

Headache, with gouty predisposition, Ferr. Phos. alternated with Nat. Sulph.

Headache, with cutting pain in left eye, and soreness in evening, Calc. Sulph.

Headache, with humming in ears, nervousness, Kali. Phos.

Headache, when heat relieves and cold makes worse, Mag. Phos.

Headache, worse from 10 A. M. to 3 P. M., Nat. Mur.

Headache, accompanied by acid risings, or vomiting sour, watery fluids, Nat. Phos.

Headache, accompanied by bad breath, Kali. Phos.

Headache, accompanied by biliousness, Nat. Sulph.

Headache, accompanied by chills up and down spine, Mag. Phos.

Headache, accompanied by chilliness, Silica.

Headache, accompanied by cold feeling in head, and cold to touch, Calc. Phos. alternated with Ferr. Phos.

Headache, accompanied by confusion, Kali. Mur.

Headache, accompanied by constipation, Nat. Mur.

Headache, accompanied by creeping coldness and numbness of head, Calc. Phos.

Headache, accompanied by diarrhea, dullness, Calc. Phos.

Headache, accompanied by drowsiness and unrefreshing sleep, Nat. Mur.

Headache, accompanied by eructations and sour vomiting, Nat. Phos.

Headache, accompanied by excessive saliva, Nat. Mur.

Headache, accompanied by flushed face, Nat. Mur.

Headache, accompanied by frothy coating on tongue, Nat. Mur.

Headache, accompanied by giddiness, vertigo, etc., Nat. Sulph.

Headache, accompanied by heaviness in limbs, Silica.

Headache, accompanied by hot, red face, vomiting of food, Ferr. Phos., Nat. Mur.

Headache, accompanied by hysteria, Kali. Phos.

Headache, accompanied by inability for thought, Kali. Phos.

Headache, accompanied by intermittent and spasmodic pains, Mag. Phos.

Headache, accompanied by loss of strength, Kali. Phos.

Headache, accompanied by lumps on scalp, Silica. ·

Headache, accompanied by nausea all afternoon, better in evening, Calc. Fluor.

Headache, accompanied by pain in temples, Ferr. Phos., Nat. Phos.

Headache, accompanied by pain over eye, Ferr. Phos.,

Headache, accompanied by pain in stomach, Nat. Phos.

Headache, accompanied by pain on top of head, Ferr. Phos.

Headache, accompanied by profusion of tears, Nat. Mur.

Headache, accompanied by prostrated feeling, Kali. Phos.

Headache, accompanied by restlessness and nervousness at puberty, Calc. Phos.

Headache, accompanied by roaring in ears, Silica.

Headache, accompanied by rush of blood to head, Ferr. Phos.

Headache, accompanied by sharp, shooting pains, Mag. Phos.

Headache, accompanied by sharp pain from back to front, on stooping, Ferr. Phos.

Headache, accompanied by sluggish liver, white or gray-white tongue, hawking or vomiting milk-white mucous, Kali. Mur.

Headache, accompanied by spasmodic pains, worse from draughts of cold air, Mag. Phos.

Headache, accompanied by tearful mood, Kali. Phos.

Headache, accompanied by tongue brownish-yellow, like stale mustard, Kali. Phos.

Headache, accompanied by tongue greenish-gray, with bitter taste, vomiting of bile, Nat. Sulph.

Headache, accompanied by tongue white or gray-white, Kali. Mur.

Headache, accompanied by uterine symptoms, Calc. Phos.

Headache, accompanied by vanishing of sight, Nat. Mur.

Headache, accompanied by vomiting of frothy phlegm, Nat. Mur.

Headache, accompanied by vomiting of sour, transparent fluids, Nat. Phos.

Headache, accompanied by vomiting of white phlegm, Kali. Mur.

Headache, accompanied by watery eyes and nose, Nat. Mur.

Headache, accompanied by weariness, yawning and stretching, Kali. Phos.

Headache, accompanied by weary, empty feeling at pit of stomach, Kali. Phos.

Headache, aggravated by laughing, Nat. Mur.

Headache, aggravated by mental work, Calc. Phos.

Headache, aggravated by any motion, Ferr. Phos., Nat. Mur., Silica.

Headache, aggravated by noise, Kali. Phos., Silica.

Headache, aggravated in evening or heated room, Kali. Sulph.

Headache, aggravated when alone, Kali. Phos.

Headache, relieved by nose-bleed, frontal, Ferr. Phos.

Headache, relieved by bandaging tightly, Silica.

Headache, relieved by cold washings, Calc. Phos.

Headache, relieved by cool air, Kali. Sulph.

Headache, relieved by gentle motion and cheerful excitement, Kali. Phos.

Headache, relieved by hot compresses, Silica.

Headache, relieved by hard pressure, rest and darkness, Mag. Phos.

Headache, relieved by hot application, pressure, lying down, gentle motion and eating, Kali. Phos.

Headache, relieved by lying in the dark, Silica.

Headache, relieved by lying with head high, Nat. Mur.

Headache, relieved by lying down, tearing around whole head, nausea on rising, Calc. Phos.

Headache, relieved by mental occupation, Calc. Phos.

Headache, relieved by pressure and lying down, forehead and top, Nat. Mur.

Headache, relieved by sitting still, Nat. Mur.

Headache, relieved by sweating, Nat. Mur.

Headache, relieved by wrapping head warmly, terrible in evening, with shivering body, Silica.

Headache, relieved by warmth, neuralgic, Mag. Phos.

Headache, relieved in open air, rheumatic, Kali. Phos., Kali. Sulph.

Headache, relieved in evening, Mag. Phos.; nausea all afternoon, Calc. Sulph.

Headache, relieved out of doors, dull across eyes, Kali. Phos.

Headache, time of, at 10 A. M. to 3 P. M., or every other day, Nat. Mur.

Headache, time of, at 10 A. M., after suppressed ague, Nat. Mur.

Headache, time of, at 10 A M., dizzy, dull, fever, thirst, relieved by sweating, and in open air. Nat. Mur.

Headache, time of, at night, with vomiting, Silica.

Headache, time of, at night or morning, boring in right temple, after buining in stomach, bitter taste and lassitude, Nat. Sulph.

Headache, time of, at night, pressive, throbbing heart, giddy, cannot remember present locality, Silica.

Headache, time of, after sunset, forehead and top, Nat. Mur.

Headache, time of, after child-birth, irregularly, Mag. Phos.

Headache, time of, during menses, heat and pressure on top, Nat. Sulph.

Headache, time of, with profuse menses, dull, heavy on top, Ferr. Phos.

Headache, time of, with menses of school girls, burning on top, Nat. Mur.

Headache, time of, with menses excessive, nervous headache, with oversensitiveness to noise, Kali. Phos.

Headache, time of, with and after menses, face red, nausea and vomiting, Nat. Mur.

Headache, time of, during and after sneezing, Nat. Mur.

Headache, time of, during stools, burning in forehead, Kali. Phos.

Headache, time of, every seventh day, Silica.

Headache, time of, in the dark, pressure as of great weight on top, Silica.

Headache, time of, in the evening, with white tongue and dry skin, Kali. Mur.

Headache, time of, morning, on waking, on crown, Nat. Phos.

Headache, time of, morning, dull, heavy, Nat. Mur.

Headache, time of, morning, from rich food, Nat. Mur.

Headache, time of, morning, on waking, Kali. Phos.

Headache, time of, morning, with weight and throbbing, Nat. Mur.

Headache, time of, morning, with chilliness and nausea, Silica.

Headache, time of, morning, with pressure in eyes, neck and back head, Silica.

Headache, time of, sunrise to sunset, worse at noon, right eye congested, worse from light, Nat. Mur.

Headache, time of, till noon, sick headache, Nat. Mur.

Headache, time of, wakens in night with headache, Silica.

Headache, time of, while reading or walking, hot and sweats, beating in temples, Nat. Sulph.

Headache, time of, worse in morning, disappearing with sun, Nat. Mur.

Heel, aching and soreness in, Calc. Phos.

Heel, piercing, ulcerative pains in, Nat. Sulph.

Heel, pricking and stinging in, Silica.

Heel, sore pains in, Calc. Phos.

Heel, stitches in. Silica.

Hips, drawing, tearing, shooting in, Calc. Phos.

Hips, pain in, as if sprained, Nat. Mur.

Hips, pain in, extending to knee, Nat. Sulph.

Hips, pain in, relieved in certain positions for short time only, Nat. Sulph.

Hips, pain in, worse from stooping and motion, Nat. Sulph.

Hips, piercing pain in, and in abdomen and back, but only during rest, Nat. Sulph.

Hips, shooting, stitching pain, from hip bone up and down, jerking, drawing, with warm feeling, Calc. Phos.

Hips, stitch in suddenly, while walking, disappears suddenly, Nat. Sulph.

Hips, stitches in, with trembling hands, languor, Nat. Sulph.

Hips, stabbing in, after a fall, Nat. Sulph.

Hips, tearing pains in, Silica.

Jaws, aching in, Silica.

Jaws, lower, drawing pain in, painful to touch, Nat. Mur.

Jaws, right, upper, pain in, with tender, swollen gums, Calc. Sulph.

Joints, aching in, with weariness, Calc. Phos.

Joints, acute, violent pains in, Mag. Phos.

Joints, acute, wandering pains in, Kali. Sulph.

Joints, darting pain in, Kali. Mur.

Joints, drawing, tearing, shooting in, Calc. Phos.

Joints, drawing, stinging, tearing pains, worse on motion, Silica

Joints, gouty pains in, Kali. Mur.

Joints, hip, pains in, thighs and neck emaciated, Nat. Mur.

Joints, pains in all, mostly on left side, Calc. Phos.

Joints, pains in, of lumbar vertebræ, Ferr. Phos.

Joints, rheumatism of, causing chronic lameness, Kali. Mur.

Joints, rheumatism of, one after another, joints puffy, little redness, high fever, Ferr. Phos.

Joints, rheumatism of, intercurrent in all cases, Nat. Phos.

Joints, rheumatism of, red, swollen, sensitive to touch, Ferr. Phos.

Joints, rheumatism of, with acid conditions, Nat. Phos.

Joints, rheumatism of, with cold, numb feeling, Calc. Phos.

Joints, rheumatism of, with crackling and watery symptoms, Nat. Mur.

Joints, rheumatism of, with swelling, Ferr. Phos., Kali. Mur.

Joints, rheumatism of, worse at night, Calc. Phos.

Kidneys, pain over, Ferr. Phos.

Kidneys, pain, violent, in region of, when lifting, or blowing nose, Calc. Phos.

Knee, darting pain in, Kali. Mur.

Knee, drawing pain in, when sitting, Nat. Mur.

Knee, gnawing pain in, tightness, Nat. Mur.

Knee, pains above, Calc. Phos.

Knee, pains, as if sprained, sore when walking, Calc. Phos., Nat. Mur.

Knee, pain in, from a blow, Calc. Sulph.

Knee, pain in, as if tightly bound, Silica.

Knee, pain in, during first few steps, after sitting, Kali. Phos.

Knee, pain, severe, shooting down legs, high fever, sleepless, Ferr. Phos.

Knee, stinging, lancinating pain, Calc. Sulph., Nat. Mur., Silica.

Knee, stitches in, Nat. Mur., Calc. Sulph., Silica.

Knee, tearing in, while sitting, stops on motion, Silica.

Knee, violent pains, below the hollow, Calc. Phos.

Knees to feet, severe, worse at night, Silica.

Larynx, pain on both sides, with hoarseness, Nat. Mur.

Lightning-like attacks of pain, gradually becoming more frequent, Kali. Mur.

Lightning-like pains along course of nerve, better from warmth, worse on right side, and when body gets cold, Mag. Phos.

Limbs, aching in, with weariness, Calc. Phos.

Limbs, flying pains, after getting wet, Calc. Phos.

Limbs, neuralgia of, Mag. Phos . Nat. Phos.

Limbs, neuralgia of, worse in evening. Kali. Sulph.

Limbs, nightly pain in, ulcers on, Silica.

Limbs, obstinate pains in, worse in changing weather, or after a cold, Silica.

Limbs, one painful, and the other numb, Silica.

Limbs, pain, after least exertion, Nat. Mur.

Limbs, pain, as if beaten, Silica.

Limbs, pain, damp weather, Calc. Phos.

Limbs, pain, during rest, Kali. Phos.

Limbs, pains, shooting down from loins, Silica.

Limbs, pain, worse at night, Calc. Phos.

Liver, pain, bursting, cutting, Nat. Sulph.

Liver, pain in, when breathing deeply, Nat. Sulph.

Liver, pain in region of and under right shoulder blade. Kali. Mur.

Liver, pain, pressive in region of, Nat. Mur.

Liver, pain, severe in region of, Calc. Sulph.

Liver, pain, sharp, shooting in, Nat. Sulph.

Liver, pain, tensive, better after passing wind, Kali, Mur.

Lung, obstinate pain in lower left, Calc. Phos.

Lung, stitching pain in right, extending through to back, Silica.

Nails, tingling, ulcerative pains in roots of, Nat. Sulph.

Navel, aching, soreness and pain around, less after passing wind, Calc. Phos.

Navel, cutting pain in region of, through to back, Silica.

Neck, boring pains in nape of, Mag. Phos.

Neck, cramp-like pains in, first on one side, then the other, Calc. Phos.

Neck, crick in, Ferr. Phos.

Neck, pain across back of, Calc. Sulph.

Neck, pain in nape, following pain in loins, Silica.

Neck, pain in nape, severe, worse at night, Calc. Phos.

Neck, pain in sides of throat, ache on pressure up to the ear, or from ear to shoulder, worse on turning neck, or swallowing, Calc. Fluor.

Neck, painful stiffness, Nat. Mur.

Neck, remittent pains in, Mag. Phos.

Neck, rheumatic stiffness or pain, dull head, caused by drafts, Calc. Phos.

Neck, stitches in, and back of head, Nat. Mur.

Neck, violent pains in back of, and in head, Nat. Sulph.

Neuralgia, as if a nail were driven, Ferr. Phos.

Neuralgia, better from pleasant excitement, or gentle motion, Kali. Phos.

Neuralgia, better in cool, open air, Kali. Sulph.

Neuralgia, blinding temple pain, Ferr. Phos.

Neuralgia, darting, shooting pain, with flow of tears, Nat. Mur.

Neuralgia, deep-seated, periodical, night, Calc. Phos.

Neuralgia, drawing, lacing pain between the ribs, Mag. Phos.

Neuralgia, in anæmic, nervous patients, Kali. Phos.

Neuralgic earache, nervous, pains in and around ear, Mag. Phos.

Neuralgic pains in, with excessive tears, Nat. Mur.

Neuralgic or rheumatic face-ache, worse at night, Calc. Phos.

Neuralgia, obstinate, in improperly-nourished people, Silica.

Neuralgia, of anus, pain long lasting after stool, Calc. Phos.

Neuralgia, of eyelids, Mag. Phos , Nat. Mur., Silica.

Neuralgia, of face, Mag. Phos., Kali. Phos., Nat. Mur., Nat. Phos.

Neuralgia, of face, better in warm room, Mag. Phos.

Neuralgia, of stomach, Mag. Phos.

Neuralgia, of stomach, relieved by hot drinks, heat or pressure, Mag. Phos.

Neuralgia, of ovaries, darting like lightning, worse on right side, Mag. Phos.

Neuralgia, of teeth, Nat. Mur.

Neuralgia, of teeth, with heat and tearing in head, Silica.

Neuralgia, over eye, darting pains on exposure to air, or before a storm, Silica.

Neuralgia, periodic, with flow of tears and red conjunctiva, Nat. Mur.

Neuralgia, periodical, acute, shooting pains, Mag. Phos.

Neuralgia, pains severe, with white or grayish-white tongue, Kali. Mur.

Neuralgia, spasmodic, crampy pain, Mag. Phos.

Neuralgia, when cold aggravates or heat relieves, Mag. Phos.

Neuralgia, with congestion, relieved by cold, Ferr. Phos.

Neuralgia, with constipation, from dryness of bowels, Nat. Mur.

Neuralgia, with crawling, coldness and numbness, Calc. Phos.

Neuralgia, with crossness, irritability, etc., Kali. Phos.

Neuralgia, with depression and failing strength, Kali. Phos.

Neuralgia, with humming in ears, Kali. Phos.

Neuralgia, with lameness, numbness, threatened paralysis, Calc. Phos., Kali. Phos.

Neuralgia, with sensitiveness to light and noise, Kali. Phos.

Neuralgia, with sleeplessness, nervousness, etc., Kali. Phos.

Neuralgia, with throbbing pain, Ferr. Phos.

Neuralgia, worse at night, and in bad weather, Calc. Phos.

Neuralgia, worse in evening, Kali. Sulph.

Neuralgia, worse when alone, rising from sitting position, or from over-exertion, Kali. Phos.

Pain, from slight pressure of clothing, Nat. Mur.

Pain, more in jawbone than teeth, Calc. Fluor.

Pain, relieved by pressure, rubbing or warmth, Mag. Phos.

Rectum, burning pain in, Nat. Mur.

Rectum, constant pains in, Kali. Mur.

Rectum, cutting, jerking, dull, sticking pain, Silica.

Rectum, sharp stitches in when walking, Silica.

Rheumatism, acute, spasmodic, sharp pains, Mag. Phos.

Rheumatism, acute when shifting from one place to another, Kali. Sulph.

Rheumatism, aggravated by heat or cold, worse in changing weather, Calc. Phos.

Rheumatism, articular (relating to joints), Ferr. Phos.

Rheumatism, articular, movement increases pain, Ferr. Phos.

Rheumatism, articular, of any part, with congestion or fever, Ferr. Phos.

Rheumatism, articular, with coldness and numbness, Calc. Phos.

Rheumatism, better in cool, open air, Kali. Sulph.

Rheumatism, between shoulders, Calc. Phos.

Rheumatism, chronic, Calc. Phos., Nat. Phos.

Rheumatism, from every cold, Calc. Phos.

Rheumatism, in back, neck or limbs, worse in evening, or warm room, Kali. Sulph.

Rheumatism, in lumbar region, Calc. Phos., Ferr. Phos.

Rheumatism, of face, worse at night, Calc. Phos.

Rheumatism, of knees and wrists, Ferr. Phos.

Rheumatism, of limbs, with swelling, Kali. Mur.

Rheumatism, of limbs, worse by violent exertion, Kali. Phos.

Rheumatism, pain, relieved by gentle motion, but increased by fatigue, Kali. Phos.

Rheumatism, pain, severe, Kali. Phos. alternated with Mag. Phos.

Rheumatism, pain, shifting, wandering, Kali. Sulph.

Rheumatism, pain, violent, Mag. Phos. in hot water.

Rheumatism, with acidity, and creamy-yellow tongue and tonsils, Nat. Phos.

Rheumatism, with biliousness, worse in damp weather, Nat. Sulph.

Rheumatism, with chilliness, Nat. Mur.

Rheumatism, with excruciating, violent pains, Mag. Phos.

Rheumatism, with pain, stiffness, paralytic tendency, Kali. Phos.

Rheumatism, with profuse, sour smelling perspiration, Nat. Phos.

Rheumatism, with sharp, spasmodic pains, Mag. Phos.

Rheumatism, with watery or very dry symptoms (after Kali. Mur.), Nat. Mur.

Rheumatism, with white or gray-white tongue, Kali. Mur.

Rheumatism, worse at night, and in hot weather, Ferr. Phos., Calc. Phos.

Rheumatism, worse by heat or cold, or changing weather, Calc. Phos.

Rheumatism, worse by motion, Ferr. Phos.

Rheumatism, worse from getting wet, Nat. Sulph.

Rheumatism, worse in heated room, or evening, Kali. Sulph.

Rheumatism, worse in morning, or when rising from sitting position, Kali. Phos.

Rheumatic pains in jaw, extending to temples, stinging in, Kali. Mur., Silica.

Ribs, sore, ulcerative pain, and throbbing below last, worse from pressure, Silica.

Ribs, stitches under left, when walking outdoors, Nat. Sulph.

Sacrum, piercing pain in middle of, Nat. Sulph.

Sciatica and gout, Calc. Sulph.

Sciatica, chief remedies. Kali. Phos., Mag. Phos., Nat. Sulph.

Sciatica, chronic, contraction of hamstrings, intermittent after quinine, Nat. Mur.

Sciatica, dragging pain, torpor, stiffness, Kali. Phos.

Sciatica, great restlessness and pain, Kali. Phos.

Sciatica, gentle motion gives relief, continued exercise makes worse, Kali. Phos.

Sciatica, neuralgic or rheumatic affections of sciatic nerve, Kali. Phos., Mag. Phos.

Sciatica, no relief in any position, Nat. Sulph.

Sciatica, remittent pain in hip-joint and knee, relieved by heat, Nat. Mur.

Sciatica, spasmodic, excruciating pains, Mag. Phos., in hot water, frequently, and alternate with Kali. Phos.

Sciatica, with symptoms of gout, alternate Nat. Sulph. and Kali. Phos.

Sciatica, worse when rising from a sitting position, Nat. Sulph.

Sciatic affections, better from motion, Kali. Phos.

Sciatic nerve, affection of, which extends down back of thighs to feet, Kali. Phos.

Sciatic rheumatism, Mag. Phos.

Shins, pains in, Nat. Phos.

Shoulder, aching in, and in shoulder blades, Calc. Phos.

Shoulder, acute pain in shoulder blades, Silica.

Shoulder, pains in, at night, better by warmth, Silica.

Shoulder, pain under right shoulder blade, Kali. Mur.

Shoulder, piercing pain between shoulder blades in evening, Nat. Sulph.

Shoulder, rheumatic pains in right, Ferr. Phos., Nat. Phos.

Shoulder, rheumatic pains in upper arm near shoulder joint, Calc. Phos.

Shoulder blade, severe pain in only when walking, Kali. Phos.

Shoulder blade, shifting pains in, intercostal neuralgia, Mag. Phos.

Shoulder blade, sticking pain in right, Silica.

Shoulder blade, tearing pain under while walking, Silica.

Spine, curved, painful, Silica.

Spine, shooting in, between hips, Silica.

Spine, soreness, pressure, tearing, shooting in end of, Calc. Phos.

Spinal cord, aching in center of, Silica.

Spleen, catching and stinging in, worse from motion, Kali. Phos.

Spleen, pain in region of, Calc. Phos.

Spleen, pressure and stitches in, swollen, Nat. Mur.

Spleen, pressive pain in region of, Kali. Mur.

Stomach, aching or pressure under false ribs, Silica.

Stomach, beating pains in, with slight nausea, Nat. Sulph.

Stomach, burning, stitching pains in a few hours after eating, Nat. Mur.

Stomach, cutting pain in, Calc. Phos., Kali. Mur., Silica.

Stomach, cutting, cramp-like pains, with headache, Calc. Phos.

Stomach, dull pains in after meals, Calc. Phos.   ·

Stomach, digging and twisting in almost every morning after drinking, followed by retching and vomiting of bitter, salty water, sweat, and trembling all over, Silica.

Stomach, neuralgia of, Mag. Phos.

Stomach, nipping, griping, pinching pains at pit of, Mag. Phos.

Stomach, pain after eating, Nat. Mur.

Stomach, pain, as if a cord was drawn around, Mag. Phos.

Stomach, pain and soreness under left ribs, extends through to back, Nat. Mur.

Stomach, pain in, worse by pressure, Ferr. Phos.

Stomach, pain in, extends to liver, Calc. Sulph.

Stomach, pain, remittent, spasmodic, Mag. Phos.

Stomach, pain under left false ribs, cough, with purulent expectoration, Nat. Sulph.

Stomach, pain, with debility, diarrhea and headache, Calc. Phos.

Stomach, pressing, screwing, twisting pain after drinking, Silica.

Stomach-ache, accompanied by constipation, Kali. Mur.

Stomach-ache, accompanied by depression or exhaustion, Kali. Phos.

Stomach-ache, accompanied by excess of mucous in mouth, Nat. Mur.

Stomach-ache, accompanied by loose evacuations, Ferr. Phos.

Stomach-ache, from acidity of stomach, or worms, Nat. Phos.

Stomach-ache, from chill, Ferr. Phos.

Stomach-ache, inflammatory, pressure aggravates pain, Ferr. Phos.

Swallowing, painful, hysteria, Silica.

Swallowing, pain in tongue, fauces, pharynx, chest and stomach, Calc. Phos.

Swallowing saliva, more painful than of food, Calc. Phos.

Teeth, aching in all, Silica.

Teeth, boring, tearing pains in, worse from cold or warmth, Calc. Phos.

Teeth, boring, burning, beating pains in, Nat. Mur.

Teeth, burning and stitching in, worse at night, and from cold air, Silica.

Teeth, drawing, tearing pains from ear to throat after eating at night, cheek swollen, Nat. Mur.

Teeth, eye and stomach teeth painful, Calc. Phos.

Teeth, molars, pain when chewing, Nat. Mur.

Teeth, molars, shooting in. Calc. Phos.

Teeth, neuralgia of, Nat. Mur.

Teeth, neuralgia of, with heat and tearing in head, Silica.

Teeth, pain constantly over whole cheek and into bones of face, worse at night, Silica.

Teeth, pain in after taking cold, Kali. Phos.

Teeth, pain in cheek bones, Nat. Mur.

Teeth, pain in filled teeth, Kali. Phos.

Teeth, pain in gland under lower jaw, Silica.

Teeth, sore and painful in sockets, Kali. Phos.

Toothache, after dark and during sleep, Calc. Sulph.

Toothache, after eating, Ferr. Phos , Nat. Mur.

Toothache, after exhaustion or mental labor, Kali. Phos.

Toothache, aggravated by warm drinks, Ferr. Phos., Nat. Sulph.

Toothache, aggravated by motion, Ferr. Phos.

Toothache, aggravated in evening, Kali. Sulph.

Toothache, at night, Nat. Mur.

Toothache, better from cold, Ferr. Phos., Kali. Sulph., Nat. Sulph.

Toothache, every other day, Nat. Mur.

Toothache, from chilling feet, Silica.

Toothache, from loss of sleep, Kali. Phos.

Toothache, in upper jaw, Kali. Mur.

Toothache, inflammatory or congestive, Ferr. Phos.

Toothache, of nervous, pale, irritable, sensitive persons, Kali. Phos.

Toothache, pressing pain, Nat. Mur.

Toothache, relieved by being in open air, Kali. Sulph.

Toothache, relieved by cold applications, Ferr. Phos.

Toothache, relieved by gentle motion, Kali. Phos

Toothache, relieved by hot applications, Mag. Phos.

Toothache, rheumatic, Kali. Sulph.

Toothache, spring and summer, Nat. Mur.

Toothache, stinging pain, preventing sleep, Silica.

Toothache, throbbing, great restlessness, worse from warmth, Nat. Sulph.

Toothache, with hot cheeks, Ferr. Phos.

Toothache, with involuntary flow of saliva or tears, Nat. Mur.

Toothache, with neuralgia of face, Mag. Phos.

Toothache, with sharp, shooting pains, Mag. Phos.

Toothache, with swollen gums and flow of saliva, Kali. Mur.

Toothache, with swollen cheek, Calc. Sulph.

Toothache, with tearing, boring pain at night, Calc. Phos.

Toothache, with ulceration, Silica.

Toothache, worse from touch or pressure, Nat. Mur.

Toothache, worse in warm room and evening, better in cool, open air, Kali. Sulph.

Toothache, worse in bad weather, Calc Phos. intercurrently.

Thighs, aching and sore, as if beaten, Calc. Phos., Silica.

Thighs, pain from heart to lower thigh, Calc. Sulph.

Thighs, pricking, shooting pain in, Silica.

Thighs, pulsative pain in, Silica.

Thighs, shooting through, extends to knees or ankles, Calc. Phos.

Thighs, sharp pain in tendons on the inside, Calc. Phos.

Thighs, tearing or shooting pains in, Silica.

Thigh bone, pain in when walking or standing, Nat. Mur.

Throat, burning in, with pains from other parts, Calc. Phos.

Throat, tearing pain down, Nat. Sulph
Thumb, stitches in ball of, Silica.
Toes, constant pain in great toe, Silica.
Toes, gouty pain in great toe, Calc. Phos.
Toes, nail, cutting pain under, Silica.
Toes, pain worse in big toe when pain in heart is better, Nat. Phos.
Toes, shooting, stinging in, Calc. Phos.
Toes, stinging or tearing in big toe when standing or walking, Nat. Mur.
Toes, tearing in great toe in evening, Silica.
Tonsils, severe pain in, worse swallowing, Kali. Phos.
Tonsils, severe shooting pain to inner ear, while eating in afternoon, Kali. Phos.
Tonsils, throbbing in, Nat. Phos.
Urination, excessively painful, Nat. Mur.
Wrists, aching in, Nat. Phos.
Wrists, lame, cramp-like and other pains, Calc. Phos.
Wrists, rheumatism in, Ferr. Phos.
Wrists, stitches in at night, extending to arm, Silica.
Wrists, tearing pains in, and in ball of thumb, Silica.

TASTE.

Taste, acid, Nat. Phos.
Taste, acrid, Calc. Sulph.
Taste, bad in morning, Calc. Phos.. Nat. Sulph.
Taste, bitter, thick, white slime coughed up frequently, Nat. Sulph.
Taste, bitter in morning, with headache, Calc. Phos., Nat. Mur., Silica.
Taste, bloody in morning, Silica.
Taste, constant taste of bile, Nat. Sulph.
Taste, disagreeable, Kali. Mur.

Taste, disgusting in morning, worse from hawking, Calc. Phos.

Taste, flabby, soapy, acrid, bitter, Calc. Sulph.

Taste, foul, Calc. Phos.

Taste, insipid. Kali. Sulph.

Taste, loss of, Kali. Sulph., Nat. Mur., Nat. Sulph.

Taste, loss of, and of appetite, Silica.

Taste, of rotten eggs, Silica.

Taste, salty, sour, Kali. Mur., Nat. Mur.

Taste, salty, with loss of appetite, thirstlessness, Nat. Mur.

Taste, soap suds, Silica.

Taste, sour, putrid, bitter, Kali. Phos., Nat. Phos.

Taste, sour taste, with burning and stinging in mouth, Nat. Phos.

Taste, slimy, Nat. Sulph.

Taste, sweetish, flabby, Calc. Phos.

Taste, water tastes putrid, Nat. Mur.

Taste, water tastes badly, vomits after drinking, Silica.

Taste, water tastes badly, Silica.

SENSATIONS IN GENERAL.

Abdomen, burning in, Calc. Phos., Nat. Sulph.

Abdomen, cold to touch, Kali. Sulph.

Abdomen, feels thick, heavy, like a weight, Silica.

Abdomen, griping in, better by kneading, Nat. Sulph.

Abdomen, wall of, tingling, numb, quivering or aching, Calc. Phos.

Anus, burning in, after stool, Nat. Mur., Nat. Sulph., Silica.

Anus, burning, itching and stitches in, Silica.

Anus, constricted feeling in, during stool, Silica.

Anus, dryness and smarting in, Nat. Mur.

Anus, itching of, from Worms, Nat. Phos.
Anus, itching of, worse in evening, Calc. Phos.
Anus, pulsating warmth in, Calc. Phos.
Anus, smarting in, with diarrhea, Nat. Sulph.
Ankles, feel as if paralyzed, Nat. Mur.
Ankles, feel dislocated, Calc. Phos.
Arm, burning and itching under, Calc. Phos.
Arm, cold feeling inside, Kali. Mur.
Arm, feels numb, like needles in, Silica.
Arm, feels tired, Nat. Phos.
Arm, pricking in, with numb hands, Silica.
Arm, trembling in, Calc. Phos.
Arm, shooting through arteries, from heart, Nat. Phos.
Back, cutting and soreness over collar bones, Calc. Phos.
Back, feeling of coldness in, Nat. Mur.
Back, feeling of weight between shoulder blades, Silica.
Back, itching of, while undressing, Nat. Sulph.
Back, jerking, pulsating, throbbing, or aching in and about shoulder blades, Calc. Phos.
Back, sore, from shoulders down, Kali. Phos.
Back, sprained, lame feeling in shoulder joint, Nat. Mur.
Back, weight in, and in shoulders, with difficult breathing, Nat. Mur.
Calves, feel as if bandaged tightly, Nat. Phos.
Calves, feel too short when walking, Silica.
Cheeks, cramp-like drawing in, stinging in jaws and teeth, Kali. Mur.
Chest, all-goneness in, Nat. Sulph.
Chest, sensation of tension in, Nat. Mur.
Chest, sore to touch, Kali. Phos.
Chest, throbbing and beating in, or under the breast bone, or pressure at its lower end, Silica.
Chest, violent oppression, with palpitation, Kali. Mur.

Chest, weak, faint feeling, walking in sun, Nat. Mur.

Crawling, all over, beginning at feet, Nat. Mur.

Craving, for salt or salty food, Nat. Mur.

Ear, burning in small spot over right, very sensitive to touch, Calc. Phos.

Ear, burning and itching externally, thin, cream-like scabs, Nat. Phos.

Ear, burning and itching externally, in warm room, Calc. Phos.

Ear, burning of right lobe, bleeds when scratched, Nat. Phos.

Ear, burning, swelling, heat, buzzing, humming, ringing, roaring, Nat. Mur.

Ear, coldness and aching externally, Silica.

Ear, coldness, followed by throbbing, heat and deafness, Calc. Phos.

Ear, cracking in when blowing nose, Kali. Mur.

Ear, cracking in while eating, Nat. Mur.

Ear, feels suddenly stopped up, Silica.

Ear, feels as if something alive in, Silica.

Ear, feels as if left ear was discharging, Silica.

Ear, fullness in, Nat. Phos.

Ear, hissing sound in, Silica.

Ear, itching, aching, pricking in, mostly in left, Silica.

Ear, itching behind, Nat. Mur.

Ear, itching in auditory canal, Kali. Phos.

Ear, lobe of right, burns, Nat. Phos.

Ear, noises in, from nervous exhaustion, Kali. Phos.

Ear, noises in, with confusion, Kali. Phos.

Ear, noises in, like running water, Ferr. Phos.

Ear, opens, with loud report, Silica.

Ear, pulsations in, Ferr. Phos.

Ear, pulsations in, heart beat noticeable, Ferr. Phos.

Ear, ringing in, Kali. Phos., Nat. Sulph.

Ear, ringing in, as of bells, Nat. Sulph.

Ear, ringing in, from engorgement of blood, Ferr. Phos.

Ear, ringing, roaring, humming, buzzing in, Nat. Mur., Silica.

Ear, ringing, roaring, from rush of blood to head, Ferr. Phos.

Ear, roaring in, after quinine, Nat. Mur.

Ear, singing in, Calc. Phos., Calc. Sulph., Kali. Phos.

Ear, singing and other noises in, Calc. Phos.

Ear, singing and ringing in, Kali. Phos.

Ear, singing, itching, ringing, worse lying down, Kali. Phos.

Ear, shooting pain in left, feels as if discharging, Silica.

Eyes, burn, dim sight, aggravated morning and evening, or near a fire, Nat. Sulph.

Eyes, burn, with sensation as of sand, Ferr. Phos., Kali. Mur.

Eyes, crawling feeling in, Nat. Sulph.

Eyes, dry feeling in, Kali. Phos.

Eyes, feel drawn and stiff on motion or use, Nat. Mur.

Eyes, feel irritated, Kali. Mur.

Eyes, feel pulled back into head, Silica.

Eyes, feel sunken, Calc. Sulph.

Eyes, itch and burn, Nat. Mur.

Eyes, sensation as of sand in, Kali. Mur., Nat. Mur., Nat. Phos.

Eyes, sensitive, itch, burn and smart after use, Nat. Mur.

Eyes, smarting and pricking in, Silica.

Eyes, smarting in, Nat. Mur., Mag. Phos.

Eyes, sticking in, Nat. Mur.

Eyeball, hot feeling in, Nat. Sulph.

Eyelids, edges of, burn, Nat. Sulph.

Eyelids, feel drawn, Mag. Phos., Nat. Mur.

Eyelids, feel heavy when using them, Nat. Mur., Nat. Sulph.

Eyelids, feel hot, Calc. Phos.

Eyelids, stitches in, as from splinters, Silica.

Face, affected, side of, tender, Mag. Phos.

Face, distorted from pain and weakness, Mag. Phos.

Feet and limbs, tired, as if paralyzed, Silica.

Feet, burn, Calc. Sulph., Nat Mur., Nat. Sulph., Silica.

Feet, burning of soles, extending to knees, Nat. Sulph.

Feet, burning of side of ankle, Ferr. Phos.

Feet, burning of, with hectic fever, Calc. Sulph.

Feet, bruised feeling in first joint, Nat. Mur.

Feet, cold limbs and feet, after suppressed foot-sweat, Silica.

Feet, cold, with palpitation of heart, Kali. Mur.

Feet, feel as if made of lead, Nat. Mur.

Feet, fidgety feeling in, Kali. Phos.

Feet, icy cold. Silica.

Feet, itch and burn, Calc. Sulph.

Feet, lame and sore, hard to walk, Silica.

Feet, uneasy, constantly moving, Nat. Mur.

Feet, very tender or dry, Silica.

Fingers, burning in tips of, Silica.

Fingers, paralytic drawing in, Silica.

Fingers, tips of sore, Calc. Phos.

Gums, burning of, Nat. Sulph.

Gums, burn, smart, while eating, Nat. Mur.

Gums, upper, feel cool, Silica.

Hair, sensation of, in throat, Silica.

Hair, smarting at roots of, head hot, Calc. Phos.

Hands, burn, or are sweaty, Nat. Mur.

Hands, feel numb, or fall asleep, Silica.

Hands, itching inside of, Kali. Phos.

Head, beating and pulsating, worse in forehead and top, with chilliness, Silica.

Head, beating and pulsating, with nausea and vomiting, worse in morning and when moving, better lying with head high, Nat. Mur.

Head, beating and throbbing on motion of body, Nat. Mur.

Head, burning in, with pulsation and sweat, worse at night, from mental exertion and talking, better when wrapped warmly, Silica.

Head, burning, on top, running to toes, Calc. Phos.

Head, cold on top, Nat. Mur.

Head, cold to touch, Calc. Phos.

Head, crawlings over, cold sensations, Calc. Phos.

Head, creeping, on the top, Nat. Mur.

Head, dizziness, Calc. Phos., Ferr. Phos.

Head, dizziness, from excess of bile, yellow-coated tongue, bitter taste, Nat. Sulph.

Head, dizziness, from exhaustion, Kali. Sulph., Ferr. Phos.

Head, dizziness, from nervous causes or weakness, worse by rising and looking upward, Kali. Phos.

Head, dizziness, from rush of blood to head, throbbing pain and flushed face, Ferr. Phos.

Head, dizziness, when walking, with weakness and oppression of head and across stomach, Calc. Sulph.

Head, dizziness, with gastric derangements, acid conditions, etc., Nat. Phos.

Head, dull, heavy feeling in, in morning, Nat. Sulph.

Head, dullness in, as if too heavy, worse in morning and after thinking, Nat. Mur.

Head, dullness of, and intellect, forgetfulness and irritability (after headache), Mag. Phos.

Head, dullness of, flickering before eyes, Nat. Mur.

Head, empty feeling in, with anguish, Nat. Mur.

Head, feels and is cold, Calc. Phos.

Head, feels as if hanging by a piece of skin at nape of neck, Silica.

Head, feels heavy, Nat. Mur., Silica.

Head, feels too large, Silica.

Head, feels constricted, worse talking and in open air, better sitting or lying, Nat. Mur.

Head, feeling as if water pipes were bursting in, Silica.

Head, feeling as if hat were on at 4 p. m., Calc. Sulph.

Head, feeling as if head were falling off, Silica.

Head, forehead, dull pressure in, with confusion, Nat. Mur.

Head, forehead, feels like busting while coughing, Nat. Sulph.

Head, forehead, pressive jerking in, worse from sudden turning, stooping or talking, Silica.

Head, forehead, pressing-in feeling, worse when stooping, Nat. Mur.

Head, forehead, pressure in, worse after meals, heat on crown, Nat. Sulph.

Head, forehead, tired feeling in, or tension, Calc. Phos.

Head, fullness and pressure, worse from wearing hat, Calc. Phos.

Head, heaviness in back head, draws eyes together, Nat. Mur.

Head, heaviness in, not relieved by nose-bleed, Nat. Sulph.

Head, hot feeling on top of, Nat. Sulph.

Head, itching, and at nape of neck, Nat. Mur., Silica.

Head, itching soon after scratching, Silica.

Head, jerks and shocks in, Nat. Mur.

Head, jerk-like pressure on top head, deep, Silica.

Head, nervous sensation in, Silica.

Head, noises in when falling asleep, Kali. Phos.

Head, pressure and heat on top, Nat. Phos.

Head, pressure, as if in bone of back head. Silica.

Head, pressure over whole head, from above down, Silica.

Head, pressure over eyes, as from heavy weight, Silica.

Head, scalp, burning on top of, Nat. Sulph.

Head, scalp, burning and itching on back of, worse while undressing and in bed, Silica.

Head, scalp, cold on top on a line with ears, Silica.

Head, scalp, constricted feeling when walking, worse in open air, Nat. Mur.

Head, scalp, itching intensely in morning on waking, Kali. Phos.

Head, scalp, itching on back head, Silica.

Head, scalp, itching, with black scurf, Calc. Phos.

Head, scalp, worse after scratching, Silica.

Head, scalp, tight sensation of, Calc. Phos.

Head, skull feels too full, nausea and vomiting, Nat. Phos.

Head, shaking, vibrating feeling in, when stepping heavy, Silica.

Head, soreness of, to the touch, Silica.

Head, temples, beating in when walking, Nat. Sulph.

Head, tightness in back head, sneezing, Kali. Mur.

Head, weak, faint feeling in, and in chest when walking in sun, Nat. Mur.

Hips, bruised feeling in, and small of back, Silica.

Itching, in nose, Nat. Phos., Silica.

Itching, in urethra, Kali. Mur.

Itching, in vulva, while urinating, Silica.

Joints, boring in, worse at night, and from stretching, Calc. Phos.

Joints, cold feeling in, Nat. Mur.

Joints, elbow feels as if struck, Calc. Sulph.

Joints, feel sprained, Calc. Phos.

Joints, feel sore, Nat. Phos.

Joints, stitches in hands, fingers and wrists, Nat. Mur.

Joints, toes, drawing feeling in, Silica.

Knee, feels sprained, Calc. Phos.

Knee, lame in morning, when walking fast, or stooping, Calc. Sulph.

Knee, tendons feel too short in hollow of, Calc. Phos.

Larynx, burning in, after burning on back of tongue, Calc. Phos.

Larynx, feeling as of a small foreign substance in, Calc. Fluor.

Larynx, itching-tickling in after itching anus, caused spasmodic cough, Calc. Fluor.

Limbs, asleep, with restless, anxious feeling, Calc. Phos.

Limbs, bruised feeling in instep, Nat. Mur.

Limbs, dragging feeling from hip down, Silica.

Limbs, drawing in, Nat. Mur.

Limbs, electric shocks in, Mag. Phos.

Limbs, feel as if asleep, Nat. Mur.

Limbs, feel heavy, Nat. Mur., Silica.

Limbs, feel hot in evening, Silica.

Limbs, feel paralyzed, Nat. Mur.

Limbs, feel stiff or bruised, Kali. Phos.

Limbs, feel tired, as if paralyzed, Silica, Nat. Mur.

Limbs, feel weak or bruised, worse in morning, Nat. Mur.

Limbs, go to sleep easily, sore and lame in evening, Silica.

Limbs, lame, tired, heavy, Calc. Phos.

Limbs, lame, worse in morning, Silica.

Limbs, sensation, as of cold water poured over, Calc. Phos.

Limbs, tired, weak, restless, crawling, tingling, Calc. Phos.

Limbs, trembling of, with nervousness, Silica.

Limbs, trembling from weakness, worse on rising, better from continued motion, Nat. Mur.

Lips, burn like pepper, Nat. Sulph.

Lips, feel parched, Silica.

Lips, tingle and feel numb, Nat. Mur.

Liver, dull, heavy feeling in, after eating, Nut. Mur.

Liver, heaviness in right side, over, Kali. Mur.

Liver, stiffness or stitches in, when bending to left side, Nat. Mur

Lung, beating in small spot in left, Calc. Phos.

Lung, bruised, sore, Nat. Mur.

Lung, burning in, from below up, sometimes down, Calc Phos.

Lung, constricted, as if lungs were too tight, with burning hands, Nat. Mur.

Lung, constriction of, with spasmodic, tickling, dry cough, Mag. Phos.

Lung, constriction of, with palpitation 'of heart, Kali. Mur.

Mouth, bad odor from, in morning, Silica.

Mouth, burning in, as from pepper, dry, thirst, gums red, Nat. Sulph.

Mouth, feels dry when it is not, Nat. Mur.

Navel, burning in region of, Calc. Phos.

Navel, momentary pinching at, Silica.

Navel, sinking sensation around, or in whole abdomen, Calc. Phos.

Nose, coldness of tip, Calc. Phos., Silica.

Nose, drawing in roots of, Silica.

Nose, feels stopped up, pain in root, Nat. Sulph.

Nose, itching of tip. Calc. Phos., Silica.

Nose, loss of sensibility, dead feeling in, Nat. Mur.

Nose, loss of smell, Nat. Mur., Silica.

Nose, loss of smell, not from cold, Mag. Phos.

Nose, numb feeling of one side, Nat. Mur.

Nose, shooting pain in tip, flying to forehead, Silica.

Nose, squirming in, Nat. Mur.

Nose, tickling in, sneezing, Calc. Phos.

Nostrils, sore, Nat. Sulph.

Nostrils, stoppage of, Kali. Phos.

Numb and rough feeling in mouth and throat, Nat. Sulph.

Numbness in arm and hand, Kali. Phos.

Numbness in arm and hand, better by rubbing, Nat. Mur.

Pharynx, cold feeling in, Kali. Mur.

Pharynx, pain in on swallowing, Calc. Phos.

Pulsating, burning warmth in anus and rectum, Silica, Nat. Mur.

Rectum, burning and scratching in, during stools, Silica.

Rectum, feels like foreign body in, constant looseness, Nat. Mur.

Sacrum, feels numb, Calc. Phos.

Sacrum, lame or aching, Calc. Phos.

Sensitiveness of face, irritation at root of nose, twitching in corners of eyes, Kali. Mur.

Sensitiveness, from want of nerve force, Kali. Phos.

Sighing, depression or moaning, Kali. Phos. .

Skin, itching of, on face, Nat. Sulph.

Skin, itching of whole body in bed, Kali. Mur.

Skin, itching on soles of feet, Calc. Sulph.

Skin, itching, pricking, stinging, as from nettles, Calc. Phos.

Skin, itching, while undressing, Nat. Sulph.

Skin, itching, without eruptions, Calc. Phos.

Smarting and dryness of anus and rectum, Nat. Mur.

Spine, sore feeling down right side, then across loins and over hip, Silica.

Stomach, bloated feeling, Calc. Phos.

Stomach, boring in, as if it would be perforated, Nat. Sulph.

Stomach, bruised feeling in on pressure, Nat. Mur.

Stomach, burning in pit of, or throbbing, Silica.

Stomach, burning in, Calc. Phos., Kali. Mur., Ferr. Phos.

Stomach, burning in, extending upwards, Nat. Mur.

Stomach, burning in, with fullness, Kali. Phos

Stomach, burning in, with water rising in mouth, Calc. Phos.

Stomach, burning-pinching in on rising, better after breakfast, Nat. Sulph.

Stomach, cold feeling in, Nat. Mur.

Stomach, cold feeling in, as of a stone, Silica.

Stomach, constant thirst, but no desire to drink, Nat. Sulph.

Stomach, constricted feeling, clothes seem tight, Ferr. Phos.

Stomach, clawing feeling in upper abdomen, Nat. Mur.

Stomach, distended, heavy feeling in, Nat. Sulph.

Stomach, drowsiness after eating, Calc. Phos., Nat. Sulph.

Stomach, empty feeling in, with pressure, Kali. Mur.

Stomach, empty, gone feeling in, Nat. Phos.

Stomach, empty, sinking sensation in, Kali. Phos.

Stomach, expanded feeling in, Calc. Phos.

Stomach, faintness in, befogged feeling in head, Kali. Sulph.

Stomach, feeling as if knives running into, Silica.

Stomach, feeling of weight below breast-bone, Nat. Phos.

Stomach, full feeling in, and in chest, difficult breathing, Nat. Sulph.

Stomach, fullness at pit of, Kali. Sulph.

Stomach, gnawing sensation in, Kali. Phos., Nat. Mur.

Stomach, gone feeling in, Nat. Mur.

Stomach, heavy, and fullness in, Nat. Mur.

Stomach, heavy feeling in, Calc. Phos., Silica.

Stomach, heavy, like lead, Silica, Kali. Sulph.

Stomach, load in, after a meal, especially raw vegetables, Silica.

Stomach, pressure at pit of, Kali. Sulph.

Stomach, pressure in, as after eating too much, Silica.

Stomach, pressure in, early in morning, Nat. Mur.

Stomach, pressure in, with rapid sinking of strength and nausea, Nat. Mur.

Stomach, pressure in, with empty feeling, chilliness, listlessness, Kali. Mur.

Stomach, sore to touch after eating, Silica, Calc. Phos.

Stomach, tight feeling in, as if tied with a string, Silica.

Stomach, tightness at pit of, Silica.

Stomach, throbbing under false ribs, better after belching or passing wind, Calc. Phos.

Teeth, feel loose, burn, sting and pulsate, Nat. Mur.

Teeth, feel sore, Kali. Phos.

Teeth, feel too large, Silica.

Teeth, feel too long, Nat. Mur.

Teeth, hollow, cannot bear air, Calc. Phos.

Teeth, sensitive to cold air or touch, Mag. Phos.

Throat, burning in, Silica.

Throat, burning, pricking, suffocative, worse at night and from cold drinks, better from warm drinks, Calc. Fluor.

Throat, choking sensation in, Mag. Phos.

Throat, cold feeling in, Kali. Mur.

Throat, dry feeling, but raises transparent mucous, Nat. Mur.

Throat, feels filled up, Silica.

Throat, full sensation in, better from belching gas, Kali. Phos.

Throat, pricking in, as from a pin, Nat. Phos., Silica, Nat. Mur.

Throat, sensation in, as if it would close, Nat. Mur.

Throat, sensation as if a plug were there, Nat. Mur.

Throat, sensation of lump in, Nat. Phos., Nat. Sulph., Nat. Mur,

Throat, sensation of lump in right side of, Silica.

Thighs, drawing on inside of, Nat. Phos.

Thighs, drawing pain in, Kali. Mur., Nat. Mur., Silica.

Thighs, drawing, sticking pains in, Silica.

Toes, itching of, or between, while undressing, Nat. Sulph.

Tongue, coldness of, and in pharynx, Kali. Mur.

Tongue, slightly puckered feeling at root of, Calc. Sulph.

Tongue, soreness of, Silica.

Tongue, soreness, and burning of tip, Calc. Phos.

Torn feeling, after stool, Nat. Mur.

Urination, burning during, stitches in bladder, Nat. Mur.

Urination, burning during and after, pain in small of back when retaining urine, Nat. Sulph.

Urination, pressing-down feeling before, Calc. Phos.

Urination, smarting and soreness in vulva during, Nat. Mur.

Urination, smarting in urethra after, Kali. Phos.

Urination, soreness and burning in urethra during, Silica.

Urination, pressure in bladder during, Silica.

Windpipe, tickling in, exciting swallowing, with no relief, Calc. Phos.

SECTION 9.—MENTAL SYMPTOMS.

MENTAL SYMPTOMS.—SLEEP.—SPEECH.

MENTAL SYMPTOMS.

Absent-minded, or distracted while talking, makes mistakes easily, Nat. Mur.

Absent-minded, cannot control thoughts, Kali. Phos.

Ailments, from grief or disappointed love, Calc. Phos.

Alternately sad and excessively merry, Nat. Mur.

Anger, bad effects of, Nat. Mur.

Anger, jaundice after, Nat. Sulph.

Anxious, about the future, Calc. Phos.

Anxiety, dark forebodings, dread, Kali. Phos., Nat. Mur.

Anxious, apprehensive, despondent, Nat. Phos.

Anxious, timid, low-spirited, mind enfeebled. Nat. Sulph.

Apprehensive, fears something will happen, Kali. Phos., Nat. Mur.

Avoids company, reserved, Kali. Phos , Nat. Mur.

Awakens screaming, Calc. Sulph.

Awkward, hasty, drops th'ngs from nervous weakness, Kali. Phos.

Backwardness, Kali. Phos.

Brain-fag, with sleeplessness, gloomy forebodings, exhaustion after talking, Nat. Mur.

Brain, confusion in, Kali. Mur., Silica.

Children, cross, ill-tempered, cry and scream, Kali. Phos

Children, peevish and fretful, Calc. Phos.

Children, walk in sleep, Kali. Phos.

Delirium, with frothy tongue, Nat Mur.

Delirium, with muttering and wandering, Nat. Mur.

Delirium, in fevers, Kali. Phos.. Ferr Phos.. Nat Mur.

Delirium, low, in typhus or typhoid fever, Nat. Mur.

Delirium, quiet. Kali. Phos.

Delirium tremens, Ferr. Phos., Kali. Phos., Nat. Mur.

Delirium, picking at bed clothes, muttering, Nat. Mur.

Depressed spirits, Kali. Phos., Calc. Phos., Nat. Mur.

Depressed spirits, with lassitude, Kali. Phos.

Depressed, tearful, lively music makes sad, Nat. Sulph.

Desires to be alone, Calc. Phos , Nat. Mur.

Despondent moods, Nat. Mur., Nat Sulph., Silica.

Difficulty in remembering things, Nat. Phos., Calc. Phos.

Dizziness, Ferr. Phos.

Dizziness, when walking, with weakness and oppression of head and stomach, Calc. Sulph.

Dullness, difficulty in thinking, Nat. Mur.

Fainting, of nervous, sensitive persons, Kali. Phos.

Fatigue, mental, from reading or writing, Silica.

Fear of man, Nat. Mur.

Fears loss of reason, Nat. Mur.

Fears will come to want, Calc. Fluor., Calc. Phos.

Forgetfulness, Calc. Phos.

Frightened easily, inclined to fear, Kali. Phos., Nat. Mur.

Gloomy thoughts, Nat. Mur.

Grasping at or avoiding imaginary objects, Kali. Phos.

Grasping, with hands, and screaming, Calc. Phos.

Haunted by visions of the past, Kali. Phos.

Home-sickness, morbid activity of memory, Kali. Phos.

Hopeless, with dejected spirits, Nat. Mur.

Illusions, mental, Mag. Phos., Kali. Phos.

Ill-humored, in morning, Nat. Mur., Nat. Sulph.

Impatience and nervousness, irritable, Kali. Phos.

Indecision, Calc. Fluor.

Indifference, with stupidity, Calc. Phos.

Indifferent, fault finding, troublesome, Kali. Phos.

Indifferent, absence of feeling or emotion, suspension of moral feeling, Silica.

Involuntary sighing, Kali. Phos., Calc. Phos.

Irritable, restlessness, vexation, Kali. Phos.

Irritable, due to biliousness, does not want to speak or be spoken to, Nat. Sulph.

Intellect, obtuse, Calc. Phos., Silica.

Life, disgusted with, Silica.

Life, looks on dark side of, Kali. Phos.

Liveliness, suddenly changes to grief and melancholy, Calc. Sulph.

Maniacal moods, Ferr. Phos.

Melancholy, Nat. Mur., Kali. Phos., Silica.

Melancholy, better when walking about, Calc. Fluor.

Memory, poor, Calc. Phos., Kali. Phos., Mag. Phos.

Memory, loss of, Nat. Mur., Kali. Phos.

Memory, morbid acting of, Kali. Phos.

Mental abstraction, Silica.

Mental labor, very difficult, Silica.

Mental symptoms, relieved by nose-bleed, Kali. Phos., Ferr. Phos.

Mental troubles, from injury to head, Nat. Sulph.

Mind, wanders from one subject to another, Calc. Phos.

Mind, weak in persons practicing self-abuse, Calc Phos.

Sits still, in moody silence (St. Vitus dance), Mag. Phos.

Sleeplessness, with brain-fag, Nat. Mur.

Spasmodic symptoms and delirium, Ferr. Phos.

Stupid look, no interest in anything, Calc. Phos.

Suicide, tendency to, Nat. Sulph.

Thought, cannot concentrate, Calc. Phos.

Thought, difficulty of, Silica.

Weeps easily, Nat. Mur.

Will is weak, Nat. Mur.

Worse after disappointment or grief, Calc. Phos.

Worse in stormy or damp weather, Nat. Sulph.

SLEEP.

Sleep, awakened from by urging to urinate, Silica.

Sleep, awakens with fright, headache, sweat, thirst, Nat. Mur.

Sleep, broken by itching from pin worms in anus, Nat. Phos.

Sleep, broken by pain from flatulency, Nat. Sulph.

Sleep, broken by pain, causing difficult breathing and one-sided paralysis, Nat. Mur.

Sleep, broken by sweat on parts of the body, Calc. Phos.

Sleep, broken or prevented by lascivious dreams, Silica.

Sleep, broken or prevented by sexual excitement and urgings to urinate, Silica.

Sleep, cough during day naps, Ferr. Phos.

Sleep, crying out in, Calc. Phos., Kali. Phos,

Sleep, difficult to, after awaking, Nat. Mur.

Sleep, disturbed, worse before midnight, Calc. Phos.

Sleep, drowsiness and yawning during forenoon and at dinner, Calc. Phos.

Sleep, drowsiness all day and evening, Calc. Phos.

Sleep, drowsiness and debility in a thunder storm, Silica.

Sleep, drowsiness, but cannot sleep, Nat. Mur.

Sleep, drowsiness during day, wakeful at night, Calc. Sulph., Nat. Mur.

Sleep, drowsiness, with bilious symptoms, before jaundice, Nat. Sulph.

Sleep, drowsiness, with gloom, headache, inability to think, ringing in ears, sweating face, prostration of limbs, Calc. Phos.

Sleep, drowsiness, lassitude and depression, Silica.

Sleep, dreams, anxious, causing restlessness, depression in morning, Ferr. Phos.

Sleep, dreams, anxious towards morning, restless, depressed breathing, Kali. Mur.

Sleep, dreams, anxious, with weeping, Nat. Mur., Silica.

Sleep, dreams crowd upon each other, Silica.

Sleep, dreams, heavy, anxious, frightful, Nat. Sulph.

Sleep, dreams, of being choked by some one, Silica.

Sleep, dreams, of burning thirst, Nat. Mur.

Sleep, dreams, of fire, Calc, Phos.

Sleep, dreams, of having a convulsion from fright, awake screaming and exhausted, Calc. Sulph.

Sleep, dreams, of new scenes, with sense of danger, Calc. Fluor.

Sleep, dreams, of robbers in the house, Nat. Mur.

Sleep, dreams, pleasant, Silica.

Sleep, dreams, that absorb the thoughts long after waking, Nat. Mur.

Sleep, dreams, vivid, like a living reality, Nat. Mur , Silica.

Sleep, dreams, vivid, natural, of the death of a relative, Calc. Fluor.

Sleep, dreams, vivid, of late readings or events, Calc. Phos.

Sleep, dreams, vivid, with weeping, Calc. Fluor.

Sleep, fright-starts in, Calc. Phos.

Sleep, grinds teeth during, Nat. Phos.

Sleep, hard to wake in morning, Calc. Phos.

Sleep, headache on awaking, Nat. Mur , Silica.

Sleep, jerking of limbs during, Silica.

Sleep, lassitude after a nap, Silica.

Sleep, laughing and whining in. Silica.

Sleep, limbs twitch, shock through body when falling asleep, Nat. Mur.

Sleep, nervous trembling in, Nat. Mur.

Sleep, night sweats in, Silica.

Sleep, night terrors in, frightened and screaming, Kali. Phos.

Sleep, noises in head when falling asleep, Kali. Phos.

Sleep, picks nose during, Nat. Phos.

Sleep, prevented by chilliness, Silica.

Sleep, prevented by restless legs, Nat. Mur.

Sleep, prevented by severe pain, Ferr. Phos.

Sleep, restless, from worms, Calc. Phos., Nat. Phos.

Sleep, restless, frequent waking, with chilliness. Silica.

Sleep, rising in, and sitting about the room, Nat. Mur., Silica.

Sleep, screams in, Nat. Phos.

Sleep, starting, jerking, snoring, Silica.

Sleep, starting and talking in, tossing about, Nat. Mur.

Sleep, starting, with trembling of whole body, Silica.

Sleep, sleepiness after eating, and in evening, Silica.

Sleep, sleeplessness after excitement, Ferr. Phos., Nat. Phos.

Sleep, sleeplessness after depressing events, Nat. Mur.

Sleep, sleeplessness after worry, Ferr. Phos., Kali. Phos.

Sleep, sleeplessness, from exhaustion or lack of brain nutrition, Mag. Phos.

Sleep, sleeplessness, from nervous causes or simple wakefulness, Kali. Phos.

Sleep, sleeplessness, from tuberculosis, Silica.

Sleep, sleeplessness, with restlessness, Ferr, Phos , Nat. Sulph.

Sleep, sleepy in morning, Nat. Sulph.

Sleep, stupid in acute diseases, or from water on the brain, Nat. Mur.

Sleep, talking in, and restless, Nat. Mur.

Sleep, tired in morning, Nat. Mur., Nat. Sulph.

Sleep, trembling hands on waking, and when writing, Nat. Sulph.

Sleep, trembling over body, better during sleep, Mag. Phos.

Sleep, trembling of limbs at night, Silica.

Sleep, trembling of nerves at night, Nat. Mur.

Sleep, twitching of hands and feet during, Nat. Sulph.

Sleep, twitching of big toes, Calc. Phos.

Sleep, twitching in muscles and limbs, Nat. Mur.

Sleep, unrefreshing, from dreams of unsuccessful efforts, Calc. Fluor.

Sleep, unrefreshed after, Calc. Fluor., Nat. Mur., Silica.

Sleep, visions in, Nat. Mur.

Sleep, wakefulness, Kali. Phos., Ferr. Phos.

Sleep, walking during, Kali. Phos.

Sleep, walking during at new or full moon, Silica.

Sleep, wakened frequently by unpleasant, fantastic dreams, Nat. Sulph.

Sleep, worse lying on back, better on side, Calc. Phos.

Sleep, yawning, excessive, Calc. Phos., Kali. Phos., Silica.

Sleep, yawning, hysterical, Kali. Phos.

SPEECH.

Begins speaking with teeth closed, Mag. Phos.

Hoarseness, from cold, Kali Mur., Kali. Sulph.

Hoarseness, from over-exertion of vocal organs, Ferr. Phos., Kali. Phos.

Slow speech, inarticulate, Kali. Phos.

Stammering, spasmodic, Mag. Phos. and Kali. Phos. Begins talking with teeth clenched.

Voice, faint, weak, exhaustion from use, Nat. Mur.

Voice, hoarse, and cough day and night, Calc. Phos.

Voice, hoarse, after painting with nitrate of silver, Nat. Mur.

Voice, hoarse, after laughing or reading aloud, Calc. Fluor.

Voice, hoarse, after taking cold, Kali. Sulph.

Voice, hoarse, from recent paralysis of vocal chords, Kali. Phos.

Voice, hoarse, in morning, with much mucous in throat, Nat. Mur.

Voice, hoarse, severe, worse in morning, with chronic catarrh, Nat. Mur.

Voice, hoarse, when talking, must hawk to clear voice, Calc. Phos.

Voice, hoarse, laryngitis, from straining the voice, Ferr. Phos.

Voice, hoarse, with sensation of swallowing over a lump, Nat. Mur.

Voice, hoarse, with pain both sides of larynx, worse on right, Nat. Mur.

Voice, hoarse, with rough larynx, Silica.

Voice, hoarse, with sore throat and hacking cough in morning, Calc. Phos

Voice, hoarse, with sore throat and dry larynx, Nat. Mur.

Voice, hoarse, worse in early morning, Nat. Mur., Silica.

Voice, hoarse, unable to talk or sing, worse by either, Nat. Mur.

Voice, slow speech, becoming inarticulate, creeping paralysis, Kali. Phos.

When, under separate symptoms, different salts are prescribed for the same trouble, that one should be selected that is also indicated by other symptoms.

When under the name of a *disease* but few symptoms are given, others will be found under the *functions* or *organs* implicated.

CHAPTER V.

NATURE'S CO-OPERATIVE CURATIVES.

DIET.—PREPARED FOODS.—BATHS.—EXERCISE.—OXY-
GEN.—REST AND RECREATION.—WARMTH.—SLEEP.—
COLON FLUSH.—THERMO-OZONE BATTERY.—NUCLEIN.
—BLOOD TREATMENT (Hæmatherapy):—NUTRITIVE
ENEMA.—MY IDEAL TREATMENT.

DIET.

The influence of material substances upon the brain is strikingly illustrated by the statement, that the Arabs manipulate their hasheesh so that there are some establishments where the peculiar quality is sold that makes a man' sing, and others where the effect is to produce continuous laughter, while another preparation causes visions, either of a delightful or a horrible character, according to the quantity; and when the drug is taken at a certain strength, the fiercest and most self-ignoring homicidal tendency is developed, whence the derivation of the word "assassin" from hasheesh. The medical superintendent of an insane asylum affirmed his ability to change the mental condition of his patients in a similar way, solely by changing their diet.

The diet question, therefore, is one of supreme importance, by which is not meant either oatmeal hobbyism, vegetarian exclusiveness, nor the asceticism which denies a good thing because it pleases the palate.

It starts with the proved facts, that human foods are divisible into four groups, called respectively, protein (i. e., albuminous or nitrogenous), fats (meat and fish fat; butter, vegetable oils), carbohydrates (C. H. O., corn-starch, sugar, gums, jellies and fruit acids), and mineral salts. Each group has its own work to perform, like four mechanics building and running an intricate machine.

Mr. Protein is a man of all trades, and can do his own appropriate work or that of either Mr. Olleum or Mr. Carbo, but not the work of Mr. Salts. Mr. Olleum and Mr. Carbo can either of them do the work of the other, but not the work of Mr. Salts or Mr. Protein. Mr. Salts can do his own work *only*. It is evident, therefore, if there is to be any material deficiency in the service of these men, it is better that it should be in that of Mr. Olleum or Mr. Carbo, because there will then be a better chance to have it supplied by the others. It is further evident that any deficiency in the work of either Mr. Protein or Mr. Salts must remain unsupplied. It so happens that their work is not only of relatively greater importance than the other two, but is absolutely necessary, while that of the other two can be dispensed with to a certain extent.

Mr. Protein furnishes nearly all the frame work, the ropes, pulleys, etc.

Mr. Salts fits the parts to each other in working order.

Mr. Olleum and Mr. Carbo furnish fuel and padding.

Now, it is easy to see that if the frame work is defective, or the parts not properly adjusted to each other, the defect is very serious, while a limited lack of fuel or padding can be supplied by Mr. Protein.

Scientific investigations have settled the relative amounts of the different groups of food elements as (when estimated dry), protein 4.2, fats 1.8, C. H. O. 18. salts $\frac{3}{4}$ ounce, needed every twenty-four hours for a man at moderate work.

Females require two-tenths less in the same circumstances.

The amount of force generated by this food in the same time, expressed as heat, is 3,500 calories, a calory being the amount of heat that will raise one pound of water $4°$ F.

The proteids are albuminoids, i. e., nitrogenized substances, represented in the blood by fibrin or liquid flesh, chemically the same as the white of egg and the gluten of wheat. If, then, these are deficient the tissues waste, the gastric fluid is impaired, and the nerves lose their tone. When the fats and C H. O. are deficient the working force and resisting power of the system against cold both diminish. When the salts are deficient the material provided cannot be built together into the machine.

In disease one or more of the functions of these food elements are disturbed, e. g., in consumption, marasmus, malnutrition, and fevers, the tissues waste for want of protein. In long-continuud abstinence the fats that are stored in the system are burned as fuel, as in the case of the hibernating period of the bear, who retires in the fall sleek and fat, but wakes in the spring lank and ravenous, having consumed his stock of fat-fuel.

The fats are also stored in the system as cushions for the mechanical machinery as well as a reservoir of fuel for future emergency.

The C. H. O. group consists of starches and sugars. Sugars consist of cane or table sugar, grape or fruit sugar, and milk sugar. The last two are ready for immediate absorption, but the cane sugar must be digested.

It is the misfortune of the people that modern cookery provides a large excess of fats, starches and sugars, and a corresponding deficiency of proteids and salts. The result is that the sugars and starches are first consumed in the system, using up the oxygen of respiration and that contained in food and drink to such an extent that there is not enough left with which to transform the proteids into tissue, thus leaving in the warm blood current the easily decomposing nitrogenous substance, which becomes an immediate and constant source of disease.

A further result is a deficiency of the protein element, with its consequences as above stated.

Little more can be done in this book than to enunciate the general principles of the subject, and this can best be done in the form of separate statements without regard to direct logical connection.

Some eat themselves into disease by an over supply of nutriment. Hundreds of thousands do the same thing by the use of food disproportioned in its elements.

Thousands upon thousands slip from acute disease into chronic invalidism by semi-starvation, in which the stomach shrinks to the insufficient supply and becomes incapable of handling an adequate amount.

A certain amount of oxygen is absolutely essential to the digestion of a given amount of food. i. e., the oxygen obtained from the inspiration of seventeen cubic inches of air for each ounce of food.

Therefore, if the respiratory power is diminished, as in consumption or from any other cause, the food must be reduced to a corresponding degree.

If the food consumed is insufficient to maintain the strength, yet is all that can be digested with existing respiratory capacity, then the remedy lies not in digestants nor tonics, but in *increased respirations*.

A table of lung capacity, computed from 5,000 observations of Hutchinson and the gymnasium record of 2,300 Amherst students, is here inserted.

Height.	Males cubic inches.	Females cubic inches.	Height.	Males cubic inches.	Females cubic inches.	Amherst male students' cubic inches.
4 ft. 7 in.	126	88	5 ft. 5 in.	206	168	194
4 " 9 "	142	104	5 " 6 "	214	176	210
4 " 11 "	158	120	5 " 7 "	222	184	224
5 " 0 "	166	128	5 " 8 "	230	192	240
5 " 1 "	174	136	5 " 9 "	238	200	256
5 " 2 "	182	144	5 " 10 "	246	208	270
5 " 3 "	190	152	5 " 11 "	254	216	286
5 " 4 "	198	160	6 " 0 "	262	224	302

It is seldom that the nutritive needs of a person in sickness can be met from the ordinary table fare of the family.

If the disease be in the stomach, the proteids that are allowed should be in fluid form and the main dependence for nutrition should be placed upon the fluid proteids and the fats and starches. In severe cases enemas of fluid proteids are necessary.

If the disease be in the digestive tract below the stomach, the sugars and starches should be given sparingly, if at all, and the main reliance be placed upon the nitrogenous foods digested in the stomach.

Beef tea and the beef extracts of the market are useful as stimulants, but of no value as direct nutrients, according to Baron Liebig, Sir William Roberts, Dr. Milner Fothergill, Prof. Chittenden and others.

In selecting the food appropriate for the sick, the above principles should guide.

A list of serviceable foods is here subjoined.

In selecting from this list, or from other sources of supply, effort should be made to procure that which is chemically appropriate, and at the same time physiologically suited, i. e., agreeable to the appetite and not opposed to any personal idiosyncracy—such as constitutional aversion or uniform unfavorable effects from use.

The most convenient proteids are cheese, peas, beans, lentils, meats, poultry, fish, eggs and cereals.

The most convenient fats are butter, cream, fat meats, vegetable oils, nuts, corn and oats.

The most convenient C. H. O are starch, sugar, rice, potatoes, cereals, peas, beans, lentils, garden vegetables and fruits.

PREPARED FOODS.

AVENOLA.

Made of wheat and oats, partly digested and thoroughly cooked. Valuable as a fat-forming and flesh-producing food. Ready for use in half a minute. With milk and fruit it constitutes an entire dietary. Twelve cents a pound, or ten cents in bulk.

Battle Creek Sanitarium Health Food Company, Battle Creek, Michigan.

BEARDSLEY'S GLUTEN HEALTH BREAD FLOUR.

Designed for general use. Claims the largest amount of gluten, and to be able to sustain under physical and mental labor without animal food. Delicious to the taste. Makes sixty-five pounds more dough to the barrel than ordinary flour. Price, $5.75 per barrel, $3.25 per half barrel.

Theo. R. Beardsley's Sons, 253 Washington Street, New York.

BOVININE.

A palatable, nutritious, easily-assimilated, fluid food, made of beef and sheep blood, fruits, glycerine, and a little whiskey to preserve it. It contains the red-blood corpuscles which, when brought in contact with the mucous membrane or raw tissues, are at once absorbed and promote the nutrition. Of great value as an adjunct to a diet deficient in proteids ; as a nutritive enema, and as a local nutritive supply to wounds, sterilized sores, and irritable conditions of the digestive tract, e. g., gastritis, dysentery, ulceration of the bowels, cholera infantum, etc. Particularly needed in chlorosis, anæmia, marasmus, consumption, and all wasting diseases. Twelve ounces contain the strength of ten pounds of meat. Six ounce bottle sixty cents, twelve ounce bottle $1.00.

The J. P. Rush Manufacturing Company,

2 Barclay Street, New York City.

BROMOSE.

A nut product in malted combination with digested starch. Especially adapted to persons who cannot digest starch, but who need an increase of fat and blood. It is claimed by the manufacturers that one pound of Bromose is equal in strength-sustaining properties to one and a half pounds of bread; equal to one pound of beef in blood and tissue-making properties. It is a vegetable substitute for malted milk. May be eaten either dry, or dissolved in hot or cold water, with milk or other liquids. Put up in the form of tablets resembling caramels, thirty in a pound box. Price per pound, sixty cents.

Sanitas Food Campany, Battle Creek, Michigan.

CARAMEL CEREAL COFFEE.

Made of cereals only. Fragrant and aromatic. An excellent substitute for coffee. Delicately flavored and satisfying. Warming and comforting to the stomach. Fifteen cents a pound, 100 cups in a pound.

Battle Creek Sanitarium Health Food Company,

Battle Creek, Michigan.

CREAM OF WHEAT BREAKFAST FOOD.

Manufactured from selected hard wheat. Desirable for weak digestion and extremely palatable. Contains the same amount of proteids as ordinary white flour.

North Dakota Milling Company, Grand Forks, North Dakota. Cushman Bros. Co., Eastern Agents,

78 Hudson Street, New York City.

ENTIRE WHEAT FLOURS.

The entire wheat kernel, except the woody, outer husk. These flours contain forty-eight per cent. more of proteids than ordinary white flour, sixty-one per cent. more mineral salts, forty-five per cent. more of fat, and more than double the amount of phosphoric acid, and are the only flours that should be made into bread.

COLD-GROUND FLOUR.

The whole wheat kernel, except the outer indigestible husk, reduced to a fine flour without the use of mill-stones. Contains all the nutriment of the grain. Should be mixed to a soft dough and kneaded well. Price per barrel $10, half barrel $5.25, less than half barrel six cents per pound.

Chas. H. Hoyt's Son, 689 Broadway, New York City.

FRANKLIN MILLS ENTIRE WHEAT FINE FLOUR.

This is a golden brown or bronze, its color being from the mineral elements contained. Made from the best wheat, and warranted as represented.

As compared with the best white flour per barrel, it contains:

Franklin Mills.		White Flour.	
Water,	12.47	Water,	21.36
Fats,	2.96	Fats,	1.64
Protein,	27.81	Protein,	18.68
C. H. O.	150.98	C. H. O.	153.61
Ash,	1.78	Ash,	0.71

In the ash the relative proportions are 0.98 to 0.45.
—Prof. B. B Ross, State Chemist, Alabama.
Price, $5.50 per barrel; $2.88 per half barrel.
Franklin Mills Company, Lockport, New York.

LAFFERTY COMPLETE FLOUR.

Made of Virginia wheat, which is claimed to contain a much larger amount of brain, bone and nerve food than the Pacific coast wheats. It is claimed also that "official analysis" has shown that it contains nearly 300 per cent. more brain, nerve and blood food than any high grade white flour. We have been unable to procure the said analysis, therefore this statement must be taken upon the authority of the manufacturers. In color it is a brilliant white, with an appetizing flavor, and makes a most excellent bread. Price, $8.00 per barrel; $4.00 per half barrel.

The Whittle & Sydnor Company, Richmond, Virginia.

OLD GRIST MILL.

All the elements of the grain are retained in same proportion and purity as nature stored them in the wheat. Bread made from this flour not only contains seventy-five per cent. more nourishment than white bread, but it is nature's own remedy for dyspepsia and constipation brought on by the excess of starch in white flour bread. Price, $5.25 per barrel, 40 cents per 1-16 barrel.

Potter & Wrightington, 60 Commerce Street,
Boston, Massachusetts.

PEELED WHEAT FLOUR.

Made without grinding. Contains all the nitrogenous and mineral constituents of the grain. $9.00 per barrel, 25 cents for five-pound bag.

Health Food Company, 61 Fifth Avenue,
New York City.

WHOLE WHEAT FLOUR.

Contains fifteen per cent. pure gluten. Made by a new process. This is a slightly larger proportion of gluten than in most other flours, and in constant and satisfactory use by the thousands of Sanitarium patients. Four cents per pound.

Battle Creek Sanitarium Health Food Company,
Battle Creek, Michigan.

"For making bread from the flour of the entire wheat, take two quarts of un-ifted entire wheat flour, a little less than a quart of warm water, one-half cup of sugar (or less if desired), one-half cake of compressed or ordinary dry yeast, and·a little salt. Dissolve the yeast in part of the water, mix sugar, flour and salt, and add the'yeast and the remainder of the water. Stir well and set in a warm place. When the dough has risen to twice the original amount, stir down and put in tins for baking, allowing it to rise a second time. This bread requires longer and slower baking than ordinary white bread. This quantity makes two loaves of bread of ordinary size."—Prof. L. M. Underwood, Columbia College, New York.

Another method is: One pint whole wheat flour, one pint milk and one egg, mixed and poured into hot gem pans and baked in a hot oven thirty minutes.

FRUITS AND NUTS are not strictly prepared foods, yet they are so healthful, convenient and adjustable that a brief outline of their utility is in place.

Dr. Dupoury, of Paris, divides fruits into five classes, viz.:

1. *The Acid*, i. e., cherries, strawberries. gooseberries, peaches, nectarines, apples, lemons, oranges, limes and pineapples.

2. *The Sweet*, i. e., plums, grapes, raisins, prunes, prunels, figs, dates and huckleberries.

3. *The Astringent*, i. e., persimmons, pomegranates, cranberries, blackberries, sumachberries, dewberries, raspberries, barberries, quinces, pears, wild cherries and medlars.

4. *The Oily*, i. e., olives and cocoanut.

5. *The Mealy*, i. e., bananas, and some apples.

Not having his distribution of fruits under this classification at hand, I have ventured to make it as above.

Oranges, figs, prunes, mulberries, dates, plums, and some pears are laxative because of their relaxant properties.

1. Strawberries and raspberries are excellent for the bilious and for the plethoric and gouty. Cherries not good in neuralgia of stomach. The juiciest apples are more digestible than the mealy.

Oranges, the juice of two before breakfast, good to starve the doctors. Lemon, lime and pineapple juice good for diphtheria.

Lemon juice good for gout.

"Apples excite the action of the liver, promote sound and healthy sleep and thoroughly disinfect the mouth; also agglutinate the surplus acids of the stomach, help the kidney secretions, and prevent calculous growths, while they obviate indigestion and are one of the best preventives known of diseases of the throat."

Eight ounces of apples with twelve ounces of entire wheat bread make an admirable meal at quite moderate work. The addition of butter fits it for more active labor.

"The English medical journal, *The Lancet*, gives the case of a child three years of age, ill eighteen months, blind, covered with ulcers from head to foot, in constant pain, pronounced incurable by eight eminent physicians, put by the ninth on a diet of ripe fruits and sugar or honey. In three days began to improve, in a few more opened his eyes for the first time in over a year, and at the end of three and a half months was pronounced cured."—H. M. Poole.

Cholera infantum has been treated successfully by sending the little patients to peach orchards to live.

2. Plums prevent gout and articular rheumatism.

The grape cure for the anæmic, dyspeptic, consumptive, the bilious and the gouty. Huckleberry juice excellent in fever.

3. The astringent fruits are especially useful in looseness of the bowels.

Juice of raw cranberries, diluted, good in typhoid fever.

4. Olive oil especially useful for defects of the excretory ducts of the skin.

5. Bananas are much like potatoes in food value.

Mealy apples are richer in nutriment than others.

Fruits should be eaten at the beginning of a meal, or between meals.

According to Dr. Sophie Lepper, the English food specialist—

"Almonds, blanched, give brain and muscle food with no heat or waste. (This is a mistake. Each ounce gives 177 calories of heat.—S. H. P.)

"Apples give nerve and muscle food, but do not give stay. (They contain more phosphorus than any other fruit or vegetable.—S. H. P.)

"Figs, dried, give nerve and muscle food, heat and waste, but are bad for the liver.

"Grapes, green, water, of little food value, but blood purifying.

" Grapes, blue, feeding and blood purifying ; too rich for bad livers.

" Lemons, thinning and cooling ; not good for daily use in cold weather.

" Oranges, refreshing and feeding ; not good if liver is 'out of order.

" Pine kernels, give heat and stay; serve as a substitute for bread. ·

·" Prunes, give nerve and brain food, heat and waste ; not muscle feeding, and bad for liver.

" Raisins, are stimulating in proportion to their quality.

" Small seed fruits (fresh), are mostly laxative.

" Stone fruits, are not good for liver troubles.

·" Tomatoes, have the same effect as lemons.

" Walnuts, give nerve and muscle food, heat and waste."

Pineapples, olives and apples aid digestion.

Vegetables contain so much woody fiber that they require very strong digestive fluids and muscular contractions for their digestion, and after all they contain very little nutritive substance.

Compare, per ounce, turnips with nuts (average), parsnips with prunes, cabbage with peanuts, potatoes with rice, beets with eggs :

	Protein.	Fats.	C. H. O.	Salts.	Calories	Time of Digestion.
Turnips.....	.009	.001	.059	.010	8.	3 to 4 hours.
Nuts (average)	.163	.628	.078	.009	193.	
Parsnips......	.020	.004	.155	....	19.	2 to 3 hours.
Prunes........	.025	.005	.615	.014	76.	
Cabbage......	.021	.003	.055	.011	10.	4 to 5 hours.
Peanuts.......	.200	.320	.400	.020	155.	
Potatoes......	.021	.001	.179	.010	23.	3 to 4 hours.
Rice..........	.074	.004	.794	....	102.	1 hour.
Beets.........	.015	.001	088	.010	12	3¾ hours.
Eggs.........	.118	.102	.004	.008	41.	2 hours.

The tubers, parsnips, beets, turnips, and sometimes potatoes and cabbage often must be excluded from the dietary.

An important rule is: Articles of food should be eaten together which will be digested in about the same length of time.

The large quantity of potash salts in vegetables retards their digestion.

Fruits are digested very quickly; apples in one to one and a half hours. Hence fruits and vegetables should not be eaten together.

When sweet fruits are taken freely, starch foods should be correspondingly diminished.

'GLUTEN.

Pure gluten biscuit, eatable and not unpalatable. Fifty cents a pound.

Biscuit forty per cent. gluten, no other ingredient whatever, brittle and crisp. Can be eaten by persons with good teeth. Forty cents per pound.

Biscuit twenty per cent. gluten. Twenty cents per pound.

All these for the use of diabetics.

Battle Creek Sanitarium Health Food Company,

Battle Creek, Michigan.

GLUTEN is vegetable fibrin and casein, with sometimes a little fat, and exists as gluten cells 1-675 inch in diameter, surrounding the starchy substance of the wheat; also as free granular gluten 1-15,000 inch in diameter mixed in with the starch. It is rich in all the mineral constituents needful for the body, in fact, "is soluble mineral food."

GRANOSE is the whole wheat berry thoroughly scoured and washed, salted, twice cooked, and is in slightly browned, crisp flakes, completely sterilized, delicately flavored and palatable. Recommended for constipation, biliousness, sick-headache and indigestion; for teething babies, old persons and invalids. Fifteen cents per package.

Battle Creek Sanitarium Health Food Company,

Battle Creek, Michigan.

GRANOLA, a combined food prepared from different grains, so as to be a perfect food, partly digested and thoroughly cooked, sterilized, ready for immediate use by softening with milk, water or broth; pound for pound has three times the nourishment of beef. Fifteen cents per package.

Battle Creek Sanitarium Health Food Company,

Battle Creek, Michigan.

GRANULA.

Prepared from Genesee Valley winter wheat, twice cooked, and ready for immediate use. A concentration of all the elements of the wheat, especially adapted to failing nutrition involving the nerve structures, and for children. Keeps well if kept dry. Fifteen cents per pound.

Our Home Granula Company, Dansville, New York.

GRAPE JUICE.

Furnishes one of the most healthful forms of the C. H. O. for the sustenance of man. In Germany and France grape cures are much patronized. They consist of living almost exclusively for several weeks upon grapes freshly picked, several pounds a day being consumed at regular intervals, and nothing but bread and water besides. The small amount of nitrogenous matter supplied by this diet renders it unfit for active conditions or for long continued use, but grape juice can be advantageously combined with an otherwise almost exclusive albuminous diet in most cases where that is found necessary.

A method of home preservation is to put into a kettle with one-fourth pint of water eight quarts of grapes just ripe but not over ripe, and scald slowly, mash them, drain four to six hours, express the juice and drain again, then sweeten to taste, boil the juice fifteen to twenty minutes, skimming frequently, pour hot into heated bottles, fill full and cork tightly with hot boiled corks, seal with wax and keep in a cool place. Will keep indefinitely.

An excellent preparation known as Welch's Grape Juice can be bought of druggists or of the manufacturer. Price thirty-five cents per pint.

The Welch Grape Juice Company, Watkins, New York.

Orange and lemon juices may be preserved the same as grape juice, by using the pulp only, freed from seeds.

INFANT FOODS.

The best is, of course, the nearest like human milk, which is, as per average of analyses of Chittenden, Watts', Dictionary, Leffman, and many others, protein .022, fats. 037, C. H. O. .069, and twenty calories per ounce.

JUSTS' INFANT FOOD.

A substitute for mother's milk, prepared from superior cereals and artificially digested to a great extent. Prepared for a child of from three to six months, it gives protein .023, fats .026, C. H. O. .049, calories 15. per ounce.

Justs' Food Company, 338 West Fayette Street, .

Syracuse, New York.

ESKAY'S ALBUMENIZED FOOD.

Made of cereals and the white of egg. Prepared with very rich milk, gives protein .017, fats .041, C. H. O. not given, per ounce.

Smith, Kline & French Company,

Philadelphia, Pennsylvania.

LACTATED FOOD.

Prepared for use as follows: Lactated food five-eighths ounce, milk four ounces, cream two ounces, water ten ounces, gives protein .015, fats .041, C. H. O. .043, calories 17. per ounce.

Wells, Richardson & Company, Burlington, Vermont.

MELLIN'S FOOD.

A cereal preparation having its starch predigested into maltose and entirely free from cane sugar.

To be mixed with cow's milk, and then gives the following analysis: protein .044, fats .030, C. H. O. .068, calories 21. per ounce.

Doliber-Goodale Company, Boston, Massachusetts.

MILK SUBSTITUTE.

Made of cow's milk one-half pint, water one-half pint, cream two ounces, Fairchild's peptogenic milk powders four measures. Entirely free from starch, and the sweet supplied by sugar of milk. Gives following analysis: Protein .020, fats .045, C. H. O. .070, calories 26. per ounce. Fairchild Bros. & Foster, New York.

CONDENSED MILK (Sweet).

One ounce, water one ounce, cream one and one-half ounces. Good for transient use, but contains too much cane sugar, and for a steady diet needs the addition of fruit carbohydrates by the time the child is four months old. Per ounce, protein .016, fats .041, C. H. O. .034, calories, 16.

ANTI-SCORBUTIC FOOD.

For young infants. Milk two ounces, cream one-half ounce, sugar of milk one-quarter ounce, lime water two and one-quarter ounces. Yields per ounce: Protein .017, fats .040, C. H. O. 070, calories 20.

SOXHLET'S FOOD.

One of the best formulas for infants' food is Soxhlets, as follows:

Two parts of milk and one part of a solution of milk-sugar of the strength of 12.3 per cent., and to each pint add six grains of sodium bicarbonate. The resulting fluid will have this composition per ounce: Casein .023, fats .024, C. H. O. .094, calories 20.

STRONG INFANT FOOD.

Whites of eggs three ounces, yolks two ounces, cream seven ounces, sugar of milk four ounces, water 43 ounces. Boil and cool the water to what will be blood heat after the other constituents are stirred in.

If desirable on account of acidity, add ten grains of bicarbonate of soda to the pint.　This gives per ounce: Protein .015, fats .042, C. H. O. 068, calories 20.

HINTS CONCERNING YOUNG CHILDREN IN SUMMER.

Bathe the child once a day in luke-warm water; if feeble, twice a day.

No tight bandaging.

Make the inner garment of light flannel.

The outer clothing light, cool and loose.

Use clean diapers always.

Give the child a bed by itself and put it in awake.

Never coddle a well child to sleep in the arms.

Never give soothing syrup nor sleeping drops.

Never give candy or cake to quiet it.

Keep in the fresh air, under shade, not in rooms heated for domestic purposes.

Give breast milk, if possible, once in two or three hours during the day, and seldom as possible at night.

Remove the child from the breast if it falls asleep.

Never give the breast when you are over-fatigued or over-heated.

If hand-feeding must be resorted to, try pure, fresh, unskimmed cow's milk.　Add to each nursing-bottle full a half-teaspoonful of sugar, and if the milk is very rich, young infants should have it diluted with one-fourth part of hot water.　Prepare the milk by filling soda-bottles to within two inches of the top, cork tightly, set into cold water on the stove and bring it nearly to the boiling point, and keep it there about twenty minutes, then remove from stove and cool slowly, set aside in a cool place.　Do not open until needed

If such milk disagrees add a tablespoonful of lime water to each bottle.

If this disagrees try pure cream diluted with three-fourths or four-fifths of pure water for a few days, then return to the milk. If this fails try some of the prepared infant's foods.

Use plain nursing-bottle with a rubber nipple and no tube, and soak both bottle and nipple, between meals, in water containing a little soda.

Do not wean the child just before or during hot weather; usually, not until after its second summer.

After six months old a little stale bread and milk may be given twice a day. After eight months old one meal a day of the yolk of fresh eggs rare-boiled.

From three or four months, slightly sweet or neutral fruits may constitute a part of the daily diet.

MILKINE.

Milkine possesses the nutritive element of milk, malt and meat. In proteids it slightly exceeds good wheat flour, while it has six times as much fat and more than six times as much mineral salts, largely lime, and the starch is all changed to sugar.

Recommended for insomnia, nervous prostration, pneumonia, typhoid fever and other wasting diseases, vomiting, and for nursing mothers. Adult meal, one to two tablespoonsful in a breakfast cup of hot water. Price, 50 cents and $1.00.

The Dry Extract Company, Janesville, Wisconsin.

MOSQUERA'S BEEF JELLY.

All the nutritious part of meat (53 per cent.) predigested with pineapple digestant into peptone, together with the stimulating mineral elements, made into a palatable beef jelly. Four ounce jar, $1.00.

Park, Davis & Company, Detroit, Michigan.

NUT BUTTER.

Nut butter is an emulsified vegetable fat, free from the germs contained in animal fat. It dissolves freely in water, and for this reason is more digestible than any of the animal fats or vegetable substitutes for them. It is claimed to have forty-one per cent. of vegetable fat and nearly nineteen per cent. of proteids, which is one-fourth more than beefsteak.

Recommended to all who cannot digest fats, and to increase flesh; also for constipation. Nut butter is a substitute for milk, cream and butter. Put up in sealed tin cases from one to ten pounds each, 30 cents per pound.

Sanitas Food Company, Battle Creek, Michigan.

NUT MEAL.

Differs from nut butter in that it is claimed to have thirty-one per cent. of nitrogenous element and but forty per cent. of fat. Per pint bottle 50 cents.

Sanitas Food Company, Battle Creek, Michigan

NUTTOSE.

A thoroughly-sterilized, partly-predigested nut product, which, it is claimed, has the same composition, looks, tastes and cooks like meat. Is of the consistency of firm cheese, and when cut in slices has somewhat the appearance of cold roast mutton. Price per one-half pound, 20 cents, one pound 30 cents.

Sanitas Food Company, Battle Creek, Michigan.

OLD GRIST MILL COFFEE.

Made of the entire wheat kernel roasted and ground, and as an all-round table drink is the best substitute for genuine coffee when economy, palatability and satisfaction are the tests. Price, 20 cents per pound, 96 cups to the pound. Many prefer it weaker, 192 cups to the pound.

Potter & Wrightington, 60 Commerce Street,
Boston, Massachusetts.

PASKOLA.

Is a starch food, predigested and particularly valuable when the starches are required, yet poorly worked up by the digestive organs. Very fattening. Dietetically it must be considered as pure starch digested into maltine dextrose and dextrine. Protein per ounce .014, fats none, C. H. O. .833, calories 98. Price, $1.00.

Predigested Food Company, 30 Reade Street,
New York City.

PANOPEPTON.

Contains in solution the entire soluble digestible sub-stances of cooked beef and wheat, and therefore presents both the peptonised albuminoids and carbohydrates in a completely assimilable form. Possesses remarkably nour-ishing and sustaining powers as a food for the sick, and nursing women. Price, $1.00 per bottle.

Fairchild Bros. & Foster, Rose and Duane Streets,
New York City.

POSTUM CEREAL FOOD COFFEE.

A thoroughly healthful food drink. Consists of about seventy per cent. of the gluten of the wheat, twenty per cent. starch, and ten per cent. saccharine matter from sugar cane. Price, 25 cents per package, 100 cups to the package.

Postum Cereal Company, Limited,
Battle Creek, Michigan.

WINSOR CEREAL COFFEE.

This is a compound of pure cereals and coffee, reducing the stimulative properties of the coffee and sustaining by the nutritive properties of the cereals. Sold in air-tight cans at 25 cents per pound, 56 cups to the pound.

The McMullen-Winsor Coffee Company,
139 Lake Street, Chicago, Illinois.

UNIVERSAL FOOD.

Made from the *germs* of wheat and barley, cooked thirty hours, then dried into a powder ready for instant use.

One package of seventeen ounces, 50 cents, is claimed to have nutritious value equal to forty quarts of good milk, or sixty eggs, or ten pounds of beef or mutton, or thirty pounds of wheat. Easily digested, very fattening, bland and palatable.

Health Food Company, 61 Fifth Avenue, New York.

WHEATENA.

A breakfast cereal that can be completely cooked in one minute. Made from peeled wheat, and has all the nutriment of the grain. 25 cents for a box of thirty-five ounces.

Health Food Company, 61 Fifth Avenue, New York.

WHEATENA.

Made from wheat, excluding the woody fiber and the bulk of the starch. If this be so, it ought to be very rich in nitrogenous elements, but as no analysis is furnished, in this, as in all other cases of similar omission, our readers must judge for themselves as to the propriety of paying eight cents a pound for a bread material of uncertain albuminous quality.

Chas. H. Hoyt's Son, 689 Broadway, New York.

WHEATENA FRUIT.

A compound of Wheatena with dates, forming a delicious food. Price per pound, 20 cents.

Chas. H. Hoyt's Son, 689 Broadway, New York.

WHEATLET.

Made from choice wheat with the outer husk removed, reduced to a granular form without the use of mill stones. Non-irritating, and while hearty enough for a strong man, suits the dyspeptic stomach.

It is claimed that when used as a breakfast mush it costs less than one cent for each person. Price not given.

Franklin Mills Company, Lockport, New York.

WATER CRACKERS, OLD GRIST MILL.

Made of pure, cold spring water and Old Grist Mill Entire Wheat Flour, and nothing else.

Capt. Jensen, who lately sailed with Lieut. R. E. Perry for the far North, took 100 large casks of these water crackers among his stores.

Non-constipating, prevent dyspepsia, rich in bone and muscle food. Price, 15 cents per pound.

Potter & Wrightington, 60 Commerce Street,
Boston, Massachusetts.

WHEAT TOASTED, OLD GRIST MILL.

The toasting process effects the same change in the wheat that occurs when fresh bread is toasted, i. e., its starch is changed to dextrine, and a delightful flavor is developed. Contains all the food qualities of the grain. Price, 10 cents per pound. 24 pounds $1.92.

Potter & Wrightington, 60 Commerce Street,
Boston, Massachusetts.

ZWIEBACK.

This is made by changing the starch of the flour into dextrine and dextrose, i. e., partly predigesting it.

No. 1. is made from graham flour containing fifteen per cent. of gluten.

No. 2. is a combination of wheat and rye flour. Specially appropriate for slow digestion and constipation.

No. 3. for acid dyspepsia and painful digestion.
No. 4. made from whole wheat flour.
Price of each, 12 cents per pound.
Battle Creek Sanitarium Health Food Company,

Battle Creek, Michigan.

A home-made zwieback can be prepared as follows: Cut good, stale, light, whole-wheat bread into half slices, half an inch thick, and bake in a slow oven not less than thirty minutes, or until each slice is browned, not scorched, all the way through.

Store in a dry place, and it will keep indefinitely. Costs about three cents per pound.

All prices are as quoted in July, 1897.

CREAM.

Is not properly prepared food. yet is capable of so many uses as a special article of diet that we give it a place in this connection. It is almost a pure fat food, and its bland qualities make it of special value in infantile constipation. One-half to one tablespoonful before each feeding, sweeten with loaf sugar if not otherwise accepted.

ICE CREAM.

Made of pure, fresh cream, no starch. A valuable food in gastritis, gastic ulcer, fevers, diphtheria, tonsilitis, scarlet fever, third stage of consumption, dysentery, inflammation of the bowels.

BATHS.

The principal objects of bathing are cleanl·ness, some change in the functions of the skin, some change in the determination of the blood, some change in the temperature of the body, or part of it, or some change of functional activity. Baths are named from the degree of temperature employed: Cold, 33° to 55°; cool, 55° to 65°; lukewarm, 65° to 70°; tepid, 70° to 85°; warm, 85° to 95; hot, 95° to 110°.

Cold Baths suddenly and powerfully contract the capillaries of the surface, and force the blood inward, thus stimulating the heart and large arteries to a vigorous effort to drive it back, which, if successful, is the *reaction* which glows and invigorates. But if the vital organs be weak and the capillaries sluggish, congestions dangerous to health, and even to life, are apt to result. Cold baths should be taken in a very few minutes.

Cold baths remove *solids* from the system, by increasing respiration, increase the number of corpuscles, the amount of hemoglobin and glandular activity.

Cold *local* baths, that is, applied to one part only, in reaction draw the blood to the part in order to replace the heat lost in the bath. Taylor says that a sitting bath, the water of which has been raised two degrees by the heat of the body, has caused the absorption by the blood of the oxygen of four or five cubic feet of air, "enough to raise a half pint of water from the freezing to the boiling point, and has eliminated from the system more than a half-ounce of its solid material."

Sea Bathing is the most stimulative form of cold bathing, the invigorating effects of the simple cold bath being heightened by the saline constituents of the water and the revulsive effect of the waves against the skin, aided also by the bracing air of the shore, temporary change in food, habits, etc.

A good substitute for a sea bath is the following mixture of salts dissolved in about thirty-eight gallons of water for one bath: Ten pounds of chloride of sodium (common salt), five pounds of sulphate of sodium (Glauber's salt), seven and one-half pounds of chloride of magnesia, and two and one-half pounds of chloride of calcium.

Cool Baths, in a person of ordinary health., slightly relax the skin, impart vigor, soothe the extremities of the nerves, and abate internal blood pressure. But in prostrate conditions, the effects are the same as from cold baths.

Tepid Baths are mild yet efficient relaxants to the skin and extremities of the nerves, relieving internal engorgements and soothing the entire system. Yet they are not suitable to strong local, or general congestion, flaccidity of structures, cool surface, colliquative perspiration, threatening gangrene, or chronic weakness of vital energy (Cook). They should take ten to fifteen minutes only.

Warm Baths are stimulating and relaxing to the surface, and soothing to nervous excitability. If continued long they excite perspiration, and may cause oppression, languor and giddiness, because the internal process of heat production is retarded, elimination of solids is checked, and respiration diminished. Time thirty to sixty minutes.

Hot Baths, rarely over 100°, strongly arouse the capillary circulation by the effort of the body to return the surplus heat given to it, relieve local rheumatism and neuralgia, accompanied by partial congestion when applied locally in the form of fomentations. They are not advisable when the skin is cold and clammy, except when impregnated with the strongest stimulants, e. g., capsicum or mustard. With perspiration excessive and warm, they are of great service Hot baths are useful to restore warmth to the body in cases of profound shock, or after exposure to severe cold, but in the latter case the circulation must be first gradually restored. They should be avoided if the patient expects to be exposed to cold within a few hours.

Hot baths should not be taken except as a remedy for disease, baths of lower temperature accomplishing all that is needed for ordinary purposes. Duration five to thirty minutes.

Pack Baths consist in wrapping the entire body in a sheet wrung out of water, with blankets so enveloping him as to maintain a tepid warmth in every part, thus producing the same effects as the tepid bath, but to a far greater degree, even to the extent of promoting the absorption of internal effusions. Sleep ensues as a consequence of the general relaxation, and care must be used, for if the pack be continued too long the over-relaxation may produce inability to tone up afterward, in serious cases.

Compresses are simply cold, local packs; *fomentations* are hot. For the latter, wet from two to four thicknesses of cotton, or linen, in the water or decoction selected, heated according to the case, and cover with three to six thicknesses of dry flannel, projecting on all sides three inches beyond the wet, and bind firmly in place. If continuous heat is required, change the wet cloth frequently, without removing the dry, by lifting the dry and slipping the wet under it as hot as can be borne. In congestions the moisture is absorbed through the capillary walls, detaching the adhering corpuscles and unclogging the blood vessels.

Vapor Baths, 110° to 140°. The famous Russian bath is vapor. The early Thomsonian method was to seat the patient enveloped in blankets, in a chair set on slats across the top of a tub of hot water, into which hot bricks or stones were put.

Another method is, to generate the vapor by putting an alcohol lamp, with or without a tin of water over it, under a chair, with blankets tent-like about both. This is the *hydro-alcoholic* bath.

Another way is, for the patient to lie in bed with the clothes raised by supporting half hoops, and have the vapor conducted under the bed clothes, or a vessel of steaming hot water put under the clothes.

Another way is, to surround the patient in bed with several hot bricks wrapped in cloths, and pour vinegar or alcohol on them.

However they may be taken, vapor baths should not be continued many minutes after the face perspires freely. They are far more penetrating and powerful than sponge baths, securing a full outward flow of blood, breaking up internal congestions, and stimulating the entire surface.

In scarlatina, measles, smallpox, erysipelas, hydrophobia, chronic skin affections, colds, rheumatism, ague, flooding, acute dysentery, lockjaw, dropsy, chronic abscesses, etc., they are invaluable. The bowels should be *first* emptied by a full injection of hot water, else the contents may be absorbed and carried through the system toward the surface.

The vapor bath should not be risked in conditions of decided prostration, in heart troubles or diseases of the large blood vessels, or in internal mortification. Persons of very delicate nervous organization are liable to faint in it because of the sudden flow of blood from the brain to the surface, and they may feel prostrated for days by it.

General Rules for Bathing. Those suffering from heart disease, faint spells, or congestion of the brain, should never bathe in the surf.

Full baths of any kind should not be taken within one

hour before a meal; within two hours after a meal; when much fatigued, or otherwise exhausted; when the body is cooling after perspiration; when cold from previous exposure (except the warm bath).

The ears should be protected with light cotton plugs in surf bathing.

Should lassitude result from surf bathing, or persistent chilliness, or numbness, discontinue it and rest; also take a strong cup of coffee, but do not try to "walk it off," as that will exhaust still more. Contrary to general opinion, the *feet* should be first wet, then the head, if preterred.

In all baths, heavy shocks should be avoided. The bath should be adapted to the person. If a cold bath is recommended for a certain condition, and the patient is used to warm baths only. begin with a tepid, gradually reduce to cool, then to cold. The abuse of water by enthusiastic believers in its virtues, is as much to be guarded against as its proper use is to be encouraged.

Women should take only such baths during the last two months of pregnancy, or while menstruating, as are appropriate to their condition.

The rule not to bathe within two hours after a meal, is of the utmost importance, as many cases of fatal "cramp" are due to the plunge into cold water when the stomach contains much food.

A patient suffering from dry asthma, with cold perspiration during paroxysm, would be injured by a tepid bath.

In excessive urination with a dry skin, a tepid sponge, or vapor bath, will diminish the flow. On the other hand, a cool bath, when the skin is moist, especially with an astringent added, will increase the discharge from the kidneys when that is deficient. (Cook.)

Persons who have reached the decline of life, whether

at fifty or seventy-five years of age, should avoid chills from whatever baths they allow. (From my " Secrets of Health.")

Water may be advantageously used internally in constipation, by sipping a glass on rising. In typhoid fever by taking eight to ten ounces an hour, sterilized. In cholera by using large quantities of hot water frequently as bowel enemas. By sipping hot water, one-half to one pint, thirty minutes before meals in nearly all stomach disorders. Should be sipped, because in sipping the action of the nerve which slows the beat of the heart is abolished, hence the circulation is quickened, the secretion of the bile is also hastened.

EXERCISES.

Increased oxygenation, more rapid metamorphosis of tissue, improved digestion and sleep, and the development and augmented strength of the muscles employed, are the constitutional results of exercise.

The specific kind to be employed in any case should depend upon the particular need of the case.

In general terms, all women, except those who live by hard, manual toil, need to strengthen the muscles of the abdomen, hips and back, and thus prevent or cure the malpositions of the pelvic organs, which cause the major part of their miseries, as well as to give them the muscular strength needed for safe child-bearing.

All *nervous* debilities, dyspeptic troubles, liver complaints and pulmonary ailments in both sexes, require lung expansion and increased strength of the muscles of the chest.

All *muscular* debilities call for the *systematic* use of the muscles implicated, not for mechanical braces as a substitute for vigor of fiber.

With these principles in view the adaptation of different forms of exercise may be briefly considered.

Walking, if done with an elastic step, that swings the weight of the body from one foot to the other, is the king of all exercises for universal usefulness. But it must be *walking*, not dawdling. If even but five yards can be covered, let it be with the swing of gladness for power to move at all, and more power will be born of the moving joy.

Carriage riding, especially with a cheerful companion, at an exhilirating gait, is a valuable form of exercise for the feeble, which may be changed by a moping pace and a glum associate into a funeral effect upon the spirits and and nerves.

The Bicycle is dangerously potent for good or ill, according to the judgment displayed in its use. As a rule, scorching is but a significant euphonysm for physical damage. Race riding, with its execrable posture, is too insane an act to be even mentioned as hygienic.

Going away from home until tired, is transforming exercise into exhausting work to cover the return.

Starting rapidly, or pushing up-hill suddenly, before the respiration is quickened to correspond with the more rapid heart-beats is to invite faintness, giddiness or hemorrhage.

Riding with a saddle that irritates the perineum is the sure precursor of very troublesome, and, it may be, serious disease of the genital organs in both sexes.

Pedaling rapidly soon after a hearty meal, if done frequently, is certain to derange the circulation, and prepare the way for a thrifty dyspepsia.

Avoiding these dangers, the bicycle is a blessing to the race, particularly to the female sex.

There is little doubt that the marked decrease in the

number of female consumptives in Massachusetts during
the past six years (in 1890 it was 1055 to 1,000 males;
in 1896 it was 974 to 1,000); is owing mainly to the greater
habituation of young women to out-door sports and recreations, among which the wheel has been the chief factor.

Rowing, as a muscular exercise, gives precisely the
development of strength in the abdomen and thighs that
women need, at the same time securing the chest expansion and deep respiration which are of even greater importance.

Horseback Riding, if habitual, is an almost unmatched
exercise for both sexes. No mere machine, however perfect, can ever fill the place of a noble horse whose every
motion is a thrill of magnetism, and whose spirit is instinct
with a life that penetrates and vitalizes every nerve of his
rider.

But he must be a horse, not a hack, and horse and rider
must be in *sympathy*, so that the bounding pulses of the
one shall throw tides of magnetic vigor into the other.

Blessed are they who can thus ride.

But a "swinging gallop" only once a month or so, is
only a pleasant fiction that hides the semi-dislocations and
inconvenient lacerations that make the hardest part of the
ride the day after. Females should not indulge in such
pastimes, because they come too infrequently to strengthen
supporting muscles that they tax to an extreme and often
relaxing degree.

Golf, lawn tennis, etc., in garments that neither restrict
respiration nor impede the circulation, should be sought
when *not too tired*.

But all these presuppose quite a stock of vitality to begin with.

What can those do who are shut in, and are, perhaps,

too poor to afford any of the means of exercise implied in
the foregoing ?

We answer, perhaps not quite as well, but well enough
to reap the results of exercise in the open air.

A couch or hammock in a shady nook in summer, and
the same, or even only a chair in a sheltered corner where
the sun shines in winter, comfortably wrapped if need be
with feet in a box covered with a warm blanket, or even
with a hot water bottle, if necessary, at least two hours of
every day, may be spent in the open air, when storms do
not forbid.

While there, *exercise* by using OXYGEN as directed in
"NATURE'S CURE," the best, the most reasonable, the
most effective exercise ever devised for the general relief
of human ills.

It is very simple, and for that very reason many will be
tempted to discard it.

But *it is as mighty as it is simple*, and you, poor one,
who complain that you cannot afford to procure the means
or appliances of recovery, ought to thank God that his
Providence has brought to you at last an efficient substitute for those longed-for things.

We quote from "Nature's Cure," by H. C. Borger:
"We can breathe air into the lungs, but not oxygen into
the blood." "It is not the exertion that is beneficial in
exercise, but what is gained by exercise—circulation of
the blood and absorption of oxygen." "If the vital force
generated is dissipated in the getting, no gain is made."
"It takes at least five inspirations and exhalations to complete the" (one) "act of respiration."

Therefore, the method is:

1. Either lying down, sitting or standing, draw through
the nose as much air as will fully expand both chest and

abdomen, clap the thumb and finger against the nostrils (not pinch them) and try to force out the air against the resistance of that obstruction.   After a second or two let out the air.   Do not hold long enough to produce dizziness.

2. Then take four short, natural inspirations.   In these the oxygen is absorbed.

3. Every fifth time proceed as in 1.

4. For beginners and weak persons, one to two minutes is enough for one treatment, but it should be gradually extended to ten or fifteen minutes.

5. Two to six treatments a day.

6. Do not force the fifth respiration so as to produce sore muscles or irritate the lungs, but as much as you can without doing so

Adhere strictly to this plan.

We have not space to explain the whole philosophy of this method, but assure our readers that it is thoroughly scientific, reasonable and practically successful.

What more is required?

Your doctor does not explain why and how his medicines are supposed to cure

Take this "Nature's Cure" upon the same basis of trust, and *use* it, especially if deprived of the means to get other things ; use this patiently, perseveringly, hopefully, and our word for it, if nature *can* cure she will!   And we know that she can in multitudes of cases, when the absence of so-called drug-helps gives her a fair chance.

But do not suppose that it is appropriate to invalids only. Being one of nature's remedies, it is suited to all degrees of strength and all forms of weakness and disease.

The objection may be raised that such a slight increase of oxygen intake can do but little; but it should be remembered that the basal function of oxygen is to quicken molecular movements. The smallest article that can be seen by the naked human eye is about 1-100,000 of an inch on a side, and is composed of from sixty to one hundred million molecules.

Risteen, in his work on molecules and the molecular theory, says, that if every man, woman and child in the world *i. e.*, 1,468,000,000, were to lay down in a straight line a molecule of carbonic acid gas, the line would not be a yard long.

Prof. Wm. Crooks, of London, says, that to count the molecules in a pin head at the rate of 10,000,000 per second would require 250,000 years.

A grain of musk has perfumed a room for twenty years, and in that time must have given off 320,000,000,000,000,-000 particles.

Will the objector kindly inform us how much oxygen is necessary to effect the movements of a few millions of molecules?

REST AND RECREATION.

Why needed.—The great American nation has become nervous, dyspeptic, sexually weak, and physically degenerated, largely by the untamed spirit of drive and conquest, which is the product of its environment and history.

Three more generations of retrogression, and, as a people, we shall be the scorn of the civilized world. It is time to *halt;* and the first reformation should be on the high ground of *rest*. *Greed* must check his speed, *ambition* must take time to breathe, *competition* must ease up for a holiday.

The Incessant Grind of the busy brain needs a let-up; and it will have it, or the impinging fibers will grind each other away. This is the very point that we are deploring. The damage to the brain-fiber is reporting itself in the nerves, stomach, manhood-power, and physical stature and strength of the younger generation. More holidays, and half-holidays, a sacred rest-hour in the hum of the day, business locked into the mill, bank, counting-room, office, store or shop, when it is closed for the night, instead of being welcomed at the home fireside and transformed into a hideous nightmare in the sleep-hours!

Rest, *rest*, REST, is what we need.

Reform the Schools.—But the mandate will never be heeded until the example is set in our public schools. *Stuff*, CRAM, FORCE, is the very spirit of school boards and teachers' institutes, until the young brain takes on an habitual type of high pressure, which will be maintained later on in the business of life until the machine crashes and the untimely end is reached.

None the less imperative is Nature's call for rest.

The habit of semi-sleep-rest should be cultivated. Sit easily in an easy chair, hands folded on lap, chin fallen upon chest, eyes closed, and breathe slowly way down to the pelvic bone, minute after minute, and soon (thinking only of the deep breathing) the whole organism will sleep, consciousness only being half dreamily alert. This rest-faculty ought to be cultivated, especially by all nervous people and brain workers.

Rest One Day in Seven is a law of Nature, as well as a law of God. The observation of Sir Robert Peel, that no man can work seven days in the week without prematurely breaking down, has been abundantly demonstrated in many ways.—Secrets of Health.

Recreations.—These are any methods of employing the time, other than the habitual ones, the outcome of which is

re-creative to the vital powers. This definition excludes
all violent exercises that are more exhausting than recu-
perating ; all methods that tease the nerves into irritability ;
and all that interfere with the dominancy of good, estab-
lished habits.

As a general rule, recreation should be in the line of the
partial or total disuse of the functions and energies that
bear the ordinary strain of life, and the substituted use of
that part of the nature that can be most pleasurably employed under the circumstances.

A day off on an excursion or picnic, or fishing or hunting, if attended with constant worriment over the expense,
is not recreation.

Visiting, with a perpetual fret over the proprieties of the
occasion, is not rest.

A public dance or other entertainment where fashionable
attire destroys physical comfort, even though it please personal vanity, is not re-cuperation. For the habitual brain
worker to rush through a fiction, or any other book, is not
giving the brain cells a holiday.

For the mother to go vacationing and take all the
younger children with her, is not disusing the faculties
that are every day on the strain.

*Better have ten hours of genuine recreation than a whole
week of sham*—labeled "vacation ! ! ! "

Rests and recreations should be timed in frequency to
the running down of the energies.

Some men can go months without any beyond what
each night and Sunday afford, but others need it every
week, and many in poor health, every day. A twenty-
four-hour clock must be wound oftener than a seven-day
timepiece.

When the balance wheel begins to vibrate feebly, the

winding should come.   Better a little before, but none
should ever wait for it to stop.

The whole secret of the matter is, all the vital powers
act more vigorously under pleasurable recreation.   Hence
digestion and assimilation, secretion and excretion are
then at their best.

Therefore the true economist who finds it necessary to
employ remedies, will reinforce them with the best practical conditions of recovery, i e., all the rest and recreation that his case requires ; bearing in mind the fact, that
it is the worst of spendthrift policy to try to make the *remedies do their own work and that of rest and recreation
also.*

The general rule given as to the disuse of the regularly
hard worked faculties is all the suggestion that can profita-
bly be made of the particular kind of recreation for an in-
dividual case, it being understood that preference should
always be given to that kind which lies furthest from the
artificialities of life, nearest to nature, and calls into play
most thoroughly the involuntary processes of respiration,
circulation, digestion, assimilation and excretion.

Whenever feasible, and it can be made so much oftener
than is thought possible, camping out from four to sixteen
weeks should be the aim of every invalid.

It needs no elaborate paraphernalia.   Just a little nook
beside some lake or running stream ; a party of four con-
genial spirits, a small tent, a few unbreakable cooking
utensils, some tin crockery for the company, and for each
an army blanket, a rubber blanket, one or two changes of
undergarments, rubber overshoes, tooth-brush, comb, soap,
and two towels, needles, thread, pins and safety pins,
pocket testament, a few postal-cards if far from home, and
some hunting and fishing gear.   In the absence of a tent,

a covered wagon will answer for the females, and the men can build themselves a brush hut for the occasion. The provisioning is of great importance. Cereal coffee for ordinary use, and Java and Mocha mixed for times of special exposure, condensed milk, canned fruits and vegetables, hard-tack and crackers, entire wheat flour for pancakes, sugar, salt pork, salt and pepper, vinegar, and some preserved fruit juice, if practicable; no butter, nor other things that will deteriorate rapidly.

If any particular stomach troubles need to be provided for, that should be done for five to ten days, then rely upon the general dietary. Two square meals and a hand lunch a day, eight to ten hours' sleep, cheerfulness, fun and frolic to the utmost capacity.

Such a two or three months' life is worth more to the ailing than twice the length of time in any sanitarium on earth at five to ten times the expense.

No medicines, but a full set of Biochemic Salts for emergencies. Of course, a hatchet, matches, some loose cords, fine and coarse, a little old muslin for bandages, and a plentiful supply on the part of each of a fixed purpose to make all the others as happy as possible.

Such an outing is a dyspepsia-killer, a consumption evader, a prostration uplifter, a blue-devil exterminator, an "all-goneness" banisher, a sleeplessness conqueror, a "poor appetite" extinguisher, and an "always-ailing" revolutionizer!

There are thousands of families, spending every year hundreds of dollars for help that they would not need if well, and for doctors and drugs that make them no better, who would be completely rejuvinated by a ten or twelve weeks' trip like the foregoing.

Of course the plan is elastic enough to admit of any

desired increase in the number, but with the one absolutely essential qualification, NO CHRONIC GRUMBLER, and no TWO DISGRUNTLED ASKANCE-LOOKERS admitted on any terms.

If any special justification of this plan is needed it is found in the fact, that, when in the Crimean war, it was found necessary to put a large number of typhoid fever patients into tents, because the hospitals were full, it proved that the mortality was less, and the progress of the patients far more rapid in the tents.

The same was the experience of our own army in the war of 1861-'64.

In addition, may be cited the practice of the best insane asylum on this continent—the McLean, at Waverly, Mass —erected at a cost of $1,250,000, where " Food and fresh Air " constitute the line of treatment, as they do also at Dr. E. L. Trudeau's famous establishment for the cure of tuberculosis at Saranac Lake, N. Y.

WARMTH.

An egg can never be hatched in a refrigerator. Warmth nourishes life ; cold devitalizes. The reason is, the white blood corpuscles (leucocytes) are paralyzed by cold, so that their defensive work, in protecting from microbes, is diminished, or ceases altogether.

The only exception to this law is the law of reaction, upon which the utility of baths is based A *temporary* chill, by means of the nervous telegraphy, immediately calls for reinforcements, and they come rushing in with the blood-current that seeks to restore the balance of circulation, and that temporary influx of the defenders raises the vitality of the part.

Hence, a law of recovery is—no chill, however produced, that cannot be overcome by vital reaction, within a very few minutes at most, is ever beneficial.

It is useless to try to toughen by any such measures ! !

SLEEP.

"Tired nature's sweet restorer, balmy sleep," is a nice thing to talk about and a nice thing to have. Our physical systems are geared for a sixteen-hour run, and can only be run to the best advantage on that plan. Because the brain never recuperates except in sleep.

When worry, pain, care, greed or nervousness prolong that run to eighteen or twenty hours, something will give way sooner or later.

Eight hours for work, eight for sleep (for adults), and eight for all other things, is Nature's plan.

How to get the eight hours sleep is the great question. The requisites are :

1. Sufficient previous exercise to cause a little tire, without enough weariness to create fatigue-fever.

2. A mind willing to sleep and ready to *glide*, not force itself into it.

3. A well-ventilated room, by which is meant a fresh supply of air from an opening one inch by twenty, at least, in moderately cool weather, and a wide open window in summer time.

4. A hard bed, but not hard enough to make the bones ache, *i. e.*, a mattress of husks or hair, or better, woven wire springs covered with a blanket, and as light top covering as can be used without chill.

5. An extra blanket always within reach to draw over in the night, when the bodily temperature sinks.

6. Occupy the bed alone.

7. Lie on the right side, head slightly inclined towards

the chest, resting on a low, hard pillow, knees slightly drawn up, arms in the most easy position possible, and no hard pressure anywhere that will impede the circulation, or cause discomfort an hour or more later.

8. If the thoughts *will* run, fix them on the least interesting subject possible, and then care not a continental whether you sleep or not .

9. Should restlessness come nevertheless, get up, pour a little cool or cold water down the spine, then see-saw with a long towel thrown over between the shoulders, so as to create a friction over the spine.   When comfortably tired try the bed again.

10. If too much debilitated for this, the same principles can be applied by the aid of nurse or friend.

11. Abjure all sleeping potions.

12. Build the nervous system up to the sleep point by hygienic measures, and Kali. Phos. four to six times a day.

13. Never try to sleep with cold feet, but plunge them into cold water and jump into bed without drying.   If too feeble to secure immediate reaction, dry with a flesh brush or coarse towel after the cold plunge, or, if necessary, have them rubbed or whipped into warmth.

14. Never try to sleep when hungry, nor take a *full* meal just before retiring.

15. Never try to sleep with a guilty conscience.

16. Never work the brain hard within an hour of retiring.   If ill or nervous, not within three to five hours.

17. If loaded with care, never try to sleep until you can "cast your burden upon Him who careth for you."   .

Brain workers, users of alcoholic stimulants, large eaters, pregnant and nursing women, and rapidly-growing children need more sleep than others, ordinarily can scarcely get too much.

COLON FLUSH.

This is a system of flushing the bowels employed by the writer for several years. It originated in suggestions accompanying various clinical reports in different medical journals, and was greatly enlarged later after reading Dr. Wilfred Hall's wonderful elucidation of the benefits of his plan. In this treatment an attempt is made to adapt the quantity, temperature and frequency of the flushes to the condition of the patient. The colon is a sewer, the position and construction of which is such that it cannot be flushed out from end to end, therefore the only practicable way is to *pump it full* and cleanse by emptying. This requires from four to eight pints of fluid. The essentials are, a good bulb or fountain syringe, preferably both, with a tube eighteen to twenty inches long between the bulb and the delivery pipe. A large soft rubber catheter to be attached to the delivery pipe of the syringe. If this cannot be obtained, the ordinary vaginal pipe of a family syringe will answer. A rolled blanket for the hips, a pillow for the head.

How to take it.—If the rectum is empty, begin in any way that suits; but if it is packed, lie on back, hips on rolled blanket, shoulders to bed or floor, insert the pipe and inject very slowly, so as to soften the mass and allow it to pass away. Then, if the bowel is packed on the left side, lie on left side, hip on blanket, left breast to bed, thighs bent close to pelvis, inject slowly, retain until desire to stool is felt, then expel. Repeat, as strength permits, until all hardness is removed from the left side, then turn on back, hips elevated, inject slowly until full, rest, turn on right side, slowly fill again until desire to stool is felt, then pass it away.

Observe.—If much prostration ensues take a cup of hot

capsicum tea, or of hot coffee, either before or after, or both ; or better still, three to six grains of Kali. Phos. in a cup of hot water.

Should it be difficult to discharge the water, dissolve in it a teaspoonful of table salt, and gently knead the colon from the right groin up to just below the short ribs and across, just below the stomach, and down into the left groin.

Flushes hot enough to excite free perspiration should never be employed when the bowel contains a mass of foul matter.

In fermenting conditions, should be used with sufficient frequency to prevent the absorption of the poisonous pro-ducts into the blood-stream.   Best time is in the evening.

In simple constipation without fermentation, the best time is on rising in the morning.

Should be used regularly, not infrequently, as long as required.

When it causes discharges of mucous or slimy matter, it shows the need of frequent cleansing.

Its·immediate physiological effects are, purification of the blood, relief of congestion of the pelvic organs, and their vitalization, hence its great value in diseases of the pelvic organs.

Rules for Temperature.

Cool or cold for inflammation ; fevers without marked prostration, and as a tonic, but never so as to produce chilliness.

Tepid, to produce relaxation ; to promote absorption, and in obese conditions.

Warm, to soothe.

Hot, for antiseptic use, if water alone is employed ;

to relieve pain ; promote perspiration ; as a stimulant ; and to recuperate in fatigue.

Any temperature when used as an ant-acid or antiseptic medium for the employment of chemicals.

For the fullest exposition of this subject in any medical work, see my "Secrets of Health," published by the Orange Judd Co., N. Y., (Cloth, 576 pages ; price, $1.50.)

To anyone who can afford the luxury, Prof. Tyrrell's Cascade Treatment is said to be a great improvement upon the ordinary method of the use of the colon flush.

Price $6.00, 1562 Broadway, N. Y.

THE THERMO-OZONE TREATMENT.

The Thermo-Ozone Battery is the name given to an appliance (not an electrical battery), by which a difference of thirty or more degrees between the battery and its poles, generates an unfelt current that decomposes water and carries the ozone directly into the venous current; thus purifying the blood and vitalizing the nerves. It is also capable of carrying medicines, when placed in solution in contact with the positive pole, into the tissues adjacent to it. Its great superiority over all forms of electricity for the cure of disease (except when the cautery is necessary) has been demonstrated so often that it needs no further proof.

It is the invention of Dr. S. R. Beckwith, for many years an eminent surgeon in the West, but now living in New York city.

Its percentage of cures of difficult and hitherto incurable diseases is simply amazing.

It is run by putting the battery into cold or hot water, and its poles upon or near the seat of the disease. The current gives no sensation, costs nothing after the purchase of the battery, and is guaranteed for two years.

It is furnished by the author of this book, and instructions for its use given without further charge. It constitutes a part of our "Ideal Treatment" in obstinate cases.

NUCLEIN TREATMENT.

This consists in supplying to the system the vital material of the lymphatic glands of animals, the effect of which is immediately to multiply the leucocytes, and thus increase the protective power of the blood against disease, and also its reparative processes.

Various preparations have been made, but Proto-nuclein is the best adaptad to use by the people, and while not designed for them, except as prescribed by a physician, it is infinitely safer than the opiates, narcotics and other drugs, etc., that they so generally use.

As a substitute for this, when not readily obtainable, the following treatment is specially commended.

BLOOD TREATMENT (Hæmatherapy.)

This consists in opposing to disease such a good and sufficient blood-supply as would have prevented the disease, had it been possessed at the outset. The blood of bullocks, sheep or chickens may be used; in rare cases the blood of human beings is employed by transfusion. The treatment introduces blood, preferably mixed with salted water in various proportions according to the case, by the stomach, rectum, hypodermic injection, or by absorption from a raw surface.

In the hands of skilled physicians it is by far the most successful form of treatment ever devised, especially in such desperate conditions as advanced consumption, typhoid fever, pernicious anæmia, cholera infantum, nervousness, collaspe from hemorrhage, old ulcers, gangrene, blood poisoning, crushed or decayed bones, mangled flesh, and burns covering a large surface.

Dr. T. I. Biggs, 1690 Broadway, New York, is the chief illustrator of this system, and his address is here given solely in the interests of the readers of this book, who have failed to find relief elsewhere.

The method was not designed for domestic use, yet it is capable of very broad and wholesome adoption by the people.

Fortunately, an article is kept at many drug stores, and can be procured by all, which contains the blood of bullocks so combined with glycerine and enough whiskey to preserve it, as to make it sterile, palatable, rich in blood-cells and of immense utility as a nutriment in weakened conditions. We have no interest in naming *Bovinine* beyond the desire to help the sick.

It is really a form of Nuclein treatment, with the advantage of supplying the white blood-cells ready for immediate work, and the rich pabulum of healthy blood with which to sustain them.

In rheumatism the red blood corpuscles are diminished, therefore, the blood treatment with the Cell-Salts, especially Ferr. Phos., is indicated, together with two liters (about 67.6 ounces) of pure soft water a day.

NUTRITIVE ENEMA.

Not given as a complete treatment in itself, but as an adjunct to any of the others when necessary. Some useful ones are as follows ;

Nutritive Enemas.

No. 1. The white of an egg stirred into two ounces of of water, containing one-third of an even teaspoonful of table salt, at a temperature of between eighty and one hundred and five degrees.

No. 2. Two ounces of salted water and one ounce of Bovinine.

No. 3. Three ounces salted water and three ounces of Bovinine.

No. 4. One grain pure Papoid dissolved in one ounce of water, *i. e.*, two tablespoonfuls ; mix with six ounces of raw lean beef, chopped fine ; keep two hours at a temperature of 130 degrees. Strain through cheese cloth, and add a little boiled water. If desired, five per cent. of brandy may be added. May also be used as an embrocation when absorption is wanted.

No. 5. Two eggs, twenty grains of pepsin, ten grains of table salt, six ounces water, slightly warmed.

How Administered.

The bowels should at first be cleansed with warm water and Ivory. or some other soap of first quality. Rest a few moments, then slowly inject the enema with hips slightly elevated, and retain, if necessary with the help of a folded napkin pressed against the anus. Repeat every three to six hours.

In cases of great loss of blood, the No. 3 should be given, every two or three hours, until the system rallies, then less frequently.

In giving the enema, a large catheter should be connected with a bulb or fountain syringe. The catheter, well oiled, inserted as far as it will go without much resistance, then inject enough to distend the bowel slightly, and work the catheter in gradually eight inches, then inject the whole slowly. If there is much irritability, so that it is thrown off too soon, repeat, and, if necessary, prepare the enema with weak poppy tea instead of salt

water, or precede it with an ounce or two of elm or flax
seed tea, or witch hazel solution.

Dr. Jones-Humphreys has devised an improved appara-
tus as follows :

A small funnel, rubber tube half inch in diameter and
eighteen inches long, one end connected with the funnel,
the other with a piece of glass tubing, and joined to a rubber catheter. The catheter is inserted, the enema poured
into the funnel and allowed to work in by absorption.
The glass tubing shows the descending nutriment.

MY IDEAL TREATMENT.

When we consider the number and complexity of diseases, it should not be deemed strange that with all their
power for good, no one of the foregoing treatments is always successful, even in all curable cases, *e. g.*, the biochemic may fail for the want of germicides or organic nutriment ; germicides may fail for lack of either biochemics
or organic nutriment ; the oxygen treatment may not suc-
ceed for lack of any or all the others ; the blood treatment
may not be a success because of insufficient antisepsis and
too little oxygen.   ,

All these together may prove unavailing by reason of a
fountain of corruption in the colon, saturating the blood
with its poisons. The thermo-ozone battery may fail because of a lack of the biochemic salts or of organic nutriment.

Therefore a combination of two or more of these means
of cure is always necessary in cases that do not readily
yield to the biochemics alone. Which of these shall be
combined in any particular case must depend upon the
nature of the case, circumstances of the patient, and the
availability of these means.

PRINCIPLES OF GUIDANCE.

1. The Cell-Salts first, last, and all the time, in every disease, rejecting the preposterous assumption that fifty cents' worth will cure a disease of years' standing and that has baffled the skill of home physicians and the power of many dollars' worth of patent medicines.

2. The colon cleansed every twenty-four to forty-eight hours by natural, full, soft movements, or by the flush, except in extreme cases when very little nutriment is taken or great prostration without fecal poisoning contraindicate it.

3. Baths for cleansing and to control temperature should never be neglected.

4. Diet always to be adapted to the condition of the patient, so as to give full nitrogenous nutrition, meaning by full all the respiratory power in use can furnish oxygen to digest, also such fuel-foods (that is, fats and C. H. O.) as the nature of the case admits. This may be, preferably, sometimes fats, at other times C. H. O. either in vegetables or fruit juice, or some such preparation as Paskola, or, in extreme cases, the alcoholics, simply as foods, not as narcotic stimulants.

5. Oxygen to the full extent of the respiratory capacity, and that capacity increased by " Nature's Cure " method.

6. When the oxygen in use fails to master the germs of the disease, then resort to such antiseptics as may be most available, and best suited to the case.

7. It is presupposed that in all these, rest, sleep, exercise and recreation have their proper and methodical use.

8. As a perfectly safe, yet efficient mode of antisepsis and general systemic invigoration, the Thermo-Ozone Battery is of great utility, and may *economically* constitute a part of the *home* preparations for the treatment of disease.

In deciding upon which of these auxillaries to the Cell-Salts should be used in a given case, let the following questions be asked, without regard to the name of the disease, namely:

1. What is obviously needed to support and improve the vitality of the patient?

2. What is plainly required to neutralize and over-power the influences that depress the vitality of the patient?

3. Which of these treatments offers the needed vital support?

4. Which of these treatments furnishes the needed antagonism to the anti-vital influences?

Common sense with close observation and careful study of these treatments will be likely to give the answer that a competent physician would give.

Suppose a case of diphtheria to suddenly develop. Ferr. Phos. and Kali. Phos. will, of course, be administered at once.

Seclusion in a room stripped to imperative necessity, follows immediately upon the discovery of the nature of the disease. Disinfection by Platt's chlorides, Bromo-Chloraline or Sanitas is constant. Local antisepsis of the patient, externally, by spongings of Sanitas or Peroxde of Hydrogen, and of the throat and nose if necessary, with Hydrozone, Sanitas, or in the absence of these, alcohol as hot as it can be borne, with sufficient frequency to remove and keep off the deposit. Meantime nutriment of Bovinine, or if that is not procurable, the fresh blood of a bullock, sheep or chicken, defibrinated, *i. e.*, the clot removed by stirring with a clean stick, and the serum mixed with milk or fruit-juice and given, thirty drops to a tablespoonful of the serum every one to three hours, depending upon quantity taken at one time and age and strength of patient; frequently, if very weak, and in small quantities.

If complications arise, the cell-salt appropriate to the new symptoms is given.

As soon as the patient is removable, disinfection of the room occurs.

CHAPTER VI.

THE CO-OPERATIVE CURATIVES OF SCIENCE.

GERMICIDES—ANTISEPTICS—DISINFECTANTS— DEODORI-
ZERS —STIMULANTS—RELAXANTS—ASTRINGANTS.

The properties of germicides, antiseptics and disinfectants are substantially the same, i. e., they are fatal to
germ life, or so sterilize the media in which they grow
as to prevent their propogation. Practically the words
are used as synonymous in this book. But deodorizers
are such substances as have the power to destroy foul and
noxous odors.

The diseased conditions in which antiseptics are appropriate, and, in most cases indispensible, because they are
secondary diseases as explained on page sixty-two, are as
follows, viz.:

Asthma, abscess, anthrax (charbon), apthe, bronchitis,
bedsores, boils, burns, breasts ("gathered"), cancer, carbuncle, catarrh, catarrhal dyspepsia, chilblains, cholera
infantum, cholera, colitis (inflamation of the colon), con-
junctivitis (inflammation of conjunctiva), consumption, diphtheria, dysintery, ear discharges, empyema (a collection
of purulent matter in the chest), chronic enteritis (inflammation, beginning in the coat of the small intestines), erysipelas, eye discharges, farcy and glanders; fevers—bil
ious, hay, puerperal, scarlet, typhoid and yellow, fever
sores, felons, fetid breath, feet malodorous, fistulas, gangrene, gumboil, gonorrhea, hemorrhoids (piles), hydrophobia, inflammations, chronic injuries, lacerations, laryn-

gitis (inflammation of larynx), leucorrhea, lock-jaw, measles, milk-leg, miscarriage, mumps, peritonitis (inflammation of membrane lining abdominal cavity), perspiration offensive, pertussis (whooping cough), pharyngitis chronic, (inflammation of pharynx) pneumonia, poisoning, scrofula, skin diseases, stomatitis, syphilis, tonsilitis, thrush, tubercles, ulcers, wounds, old.

A great variety of antiseptics have been placed upon the market, nearly all of them with some merit, but some of special excellence are named in this book, together with particular adaptations in certain cases. The list is longer than would be necessary, but for the fact, few if any of them are kept in all parts of the country, and their use should not be contingent upon ability to procure any particular kind.

It is not expected that their internal use will kill all the germs of disease, for it is very doubtful whether any one of sufficient germicidal property to do that can be inocuous to the living organism. But they do sterilize the medium in which germs propagate, and thus preventing their rapid increase, the leucocytes of the blood overcome the germs.

The directions accompanying these antiseptics should be carefully studied.

ADAPTATION.

The best of remedies may be of no use or even harmful if the laws of adaptation are not studied. These laws relate to tolerance by the stomach, digestibility, non-disagreeing properties, quantity, frequency of dosage, etc. In short, everything that makes keen observation of effects better than blind following of prescription. Every person who treats himself, child or other person, puts himself thereby in the place of a physician, and is bound by the obligations of the relation to study his patient, observe the effects of everything done or omitted, and meet all *unfavorable manifestations* with such MODIFICATIONS of dosage or application as his common sense may dictate.

PRECAUTIONARY DISINFECTION.

In all run down conditions of the system, as well as in all cases of special exposure to disease, the precaution should be taken to use antiseptics in order to prevent the possible colonization of some of the many kinds of disease germs that are constantly swarming in the dust of the streets and in the air. For this purpose Listerine, Menthymos and Zymocide are especially pleasant and sufficiently effective.

Dr. Manfredi has discovered that the health of the people of Naples, Italy, corresponds with the number of microbes found in the dust of the streets. The healthiest streets had only 10,000,000 per gramme (the twenty-eight and three-tenths of an ounce avoirdupois), while the filthiest streets and most unhealthy sections had 5,000,000,000 per gramme. Among these were the microbes of pus, the baccillus of malignant dropsy, lock-jaw, tubercule and fatal blood-poisoning.

When it is expedient to disinfect and deodorize the hands, ground mustard rubbed on freely for five minutes, with corn meal and soap, and worked into all the creases and under the nails will be found an efficient and satisfactory article.

DISINFECTION DURING CONTAGIOUS DISEASES.

The laws of different States vary somewhat in their characterization of "contagious diseases," but the following are named by one or more States as such, viz.:

Asiatic cholera, small-pox, diphtheria (membranous

croup), scarlet fever, typhoid fever, tuberculosis (consumption), yellow fever, typhus fever, measles and cerebrospinal meningitis. Some foreign countries add bubonic plague, erysipelas, and relapsing, continued and puerperal fevers

In these diseases the health of the public requires thorough disinfection, which should consist of—

1. The internal use of the most appropriate antiseptic that can be had.

For *all* purposes Hydrozone is to be preferred, although in the milder forms of disease, Euthymol, Menthymos, Glycozone, Per-oxide of Hydrogen (medicinal), Listerine, Sanitas and Zymocide, may be relied upon.

Consult directions with the preparations, for dosage and modes of application.

2. Sponge the body with a solution of the antiseptic, with sufficient frequency and in such strength as to destroy the germs upon the surface.

See directions with the preparation for the strength of the solution.

3. Destroy the germicidal property of all excretions, by mixing with them hot water. two and a half gallons, copperas four pounds, carbolic acid four pounds ; or copperas ten pounds, in a bucket of water ; or sulphate of zinc eight ounces, carbolic acid one ounce, water three gallons. A teacupful for a bed-pan or chamber vessel each time it is used ; pour some frequently into the water closet. For drains, ditches and sewers, one pound of chloride of lime is sufficient for a thousand gallons of running sewage.

4. Render the air of the room antiseptic by free ventilation, the admission of the direct rays of the sun, unless the condition of the eyes preclude it, and by keeping

cloths hung in the room wet with Platt's chlorides, Bromochloralum, Sanitas, or by spraying Sanitas, or Peroxide of Hydrogen in the room. If the room has a fire-place, kindle a little fire in it two or three times a day, and keep the fire-place open. Permangate of potash and oxalic acid, each one ounce, moistened with twice the amount of water in an open vessel, will emit ozone freely, and may be used in place of the antiseptics named above.

Reduce to a minimum the possible lodging places of the germs, by striping the room of carpets, hangings, curtains, furniture, bric-a-brac, and reduce it to one small table, the bed, and one chair for the nurse, unless an inexpensive cot be allowed for changing the patient to, in order to have the bed aired and purified.

6. Disinfect all dishes and eating utensils and clothes used by or in contact with the patient, by washing the utensils in boiling water, and boiling the clothes not less than thirty minutes.

Of course, young children will have been sent away upon the outbreak of the disease, and all through the sickness a sheet moistened with a disinfectant has been hung across the door of the sick room. The article used should be the one most agreeable to the patient.

The nurse has not mingled with the family, and the loose wrapper that the mother has worn in the sick-room has not been worn about the house.

DISINFECTION AFTER CONTAGIOUS DISEASES.

By this is meant, whether the patient recovers or dies, the same care should be exercised to prevent infection by the disease germs.

1. Destroy by fire all inexpensive clothing, carpets, curtains or other fabrics, except such as are washable.

2. All washable articles should be boiled from twenty to forty minutes.

3. All beds, mattresses, bolsters, pillows, carpets, rugs, stuffing of chairs and cushions to be opened and submitted to the action of hot steam fifteen minutes.

If there are no facilities for this, then fumigate them thoroughly twenty-four hours with burning sulphur in tin cans or earthen jars placed in water or on bricks. Allow one pound of sulphur to every 1,000 cubic feet of air space (found by multiplying height, breadth and length of the room together). Cover metalic surfaces which will tarnish with a mixture of tallow, oil and whiting. Hang blankets and spreads on a line in the middle of the room. Open closets and drawers, paste strips of paper around the windows, doors, and all cracks, including the fireplace. Pour a little alcohol over each can of sulphur and light the one furthest from the door first, then the others, and hasten out of the poisonous fumes, close the door and paste strips of paper around it on the outside. After twenty-four hours open and ventilate twenty-four hours longer.

Another method is, after closing the room as above have in an earthern vessel a mixture of equal parts of common salt and black oxide of manganese, one ounce of each to every 100 cubic feet of air space. To each ounce of this mixture add one ounce of a fifty per cent. solution of sulphuric acid in water, and close the door at once for twenty-four hours, then ventilate twenty-four hours as before.

4. Wash the floor with a 1 to 1,000 corrosive sublimate solution, or with Sanitas fluid. Spray the same over the walls and into all crevices of windows, doors, etc., and wash all the furniture with it after the upholstery has been removed. *The corrosive sublimate solution is extremely poisonous.*

5. Tear the paper from the walls and burn it, and whitewash thoroughly.

6. Wash picture frames, brass and iron work, etc., with Sanitas, unless covered with the preparation previously named.

7. Leave the windows open for two days, then scrub the floors with soap and soda; whitewash again and paint.

This is thorough disinfection, because it reaches the chief sources of danger, namely the floors, walls and furniture.

DISINFECTING PREPARATIONS.

In selecting these, the object has been to secure—
1. Thorough efficiency.
2. As great economy as practicable.
3. Availability.

No doubt some excellent preparations have been passed by, but the best has been done that could be with the information at hand.

BROMO CHLORALUM.

Bromo Chemical Company, 241 and 243 West Broadway, New York city. Saline, antiseptic, alterative, styptic and germicide.

Has no odor of its own, but is a strong deodorant.

Non-poisonous. 50 cents per pint.

BROMINE is an inexpensive by-product of the manufacture of salt, selling at seventy cents a pounds, and in solutions containing one part in weight to about eight hundred of water, it may be used freely without affecting anything it may touch. A few quarts will thoroughly deodorize an ordinary house. The undiluted bromine is strongly corrosive, and if it touches the skin causes a painful burn.

CINNAMON, oil of, is a very useful antiseptic, while the powder is a valuable astringent.

Peculiarly valuable in cholera, dysintery, diarrhea, etc.

EUTHYMOL.

Parke, Davis & Co., Detroit, Mich. Antiseptic, non-poisonous. Used as a spray, or internally in doses of one teaspoonful three or four times a day.

An excellent and agreeable substitute for iodoform and carbolic acid, and equal in antiseptic power. Must not be exposed to cold. 75 cents per pint.

CHLORO–PHENIQUE.

Phenique Chemical Company, St. Louis, Mo. A chemical compound of chlorine and phenic acid. Non-poisonous, non-irritant.

Suitable for use in all cases externally where carbolic acid would be serviceable, and without its danger. One of its chief merits is its pain-relieving quality.

For burns, scalds, lacerated wounds and painful contusions it is of great value. Price, per bottle, $1.

GLYCOZONE.

Is chemically pure glycerine and ozone, not mixed, but chemically combined under peculiar conditions.

Charles Marchand, 28 Prince Street, New York Four ounces $1.00.

It stimulates healthy granulations, acts in a general way like Hydrozone, which see, but much slower. Must not be taken with any drug, nor come in contact with any metal, but be used with glass or hard rubber.

HYDROGEN, PEROXIDE OF (MEDICINAL), 15 vol. Solution.

Charles Marchand, 28 Prince Street, New York. Four ounces 50 cents.

This is a 4.5 per cent. solution of pure H_2O_2, which yields fifteen times its own volume of nascent oxygen.

Its effect is like that of Hydrozone, which see, but is only half as strong.   One of the most valuable discoveries of modern chemistry.

HYDROZONE.

Yields thirty times its own volume of nascent oxygen, aud is very nearly like ozone. It destroys vegetable microbes, stimulates healing granulations, and instantly annihilates the germs in old sores, while it has no effect upon healthy tissues.

As a germicide, its strength is—
3 times greater than bichloride of mercury.
5 times greater than nitrate of silver.
10 times greater than iodine.
24 times greater than bromine.
28 times greater than iodoform.
100 times greater than muriatic acid.
128 times greater than carbolic acid.
140 times greater than permanganate of potash.
300 times greater than boracic acid.
360 times greater than lactic acid.

And is perfectly *harmless*, while many of these are poisonous.   It is the great pus destroyer of modern chemistry. Must not be injected into a closed cavity without a vent, because its rapid elimination of oxygen would distend it painfully, and perhaps dangerously.   Should be used in such cases with a double catheter.

Charles Marchand, 28 Prince Street, New York.   Small size bottle 50 cents.

LISTERINE.

Lambert Pharmacal Company, St. Louis, Mo.   75 cents per fourteen ounces.

A fragrant antiseptic, with a germicidal potency equal

to a five per cent. solution of carbolic acid ; non-irritating and non-poisonous, and a pleasant deodorizer.

It is important to obtain it in the original package, as proved by the test purchases made by the manufacturers in 1893, of twenty-five cents worth of Listerine from each of 479 Chicago druggists. Twenty-four gave Listerine diluted with water or glycerine, and 204 gave an imitation containing no Listerine.

MENTHYMOS.

Fragrant, harmless, equal in antiseptic power to Listerine, Euthymol or Zymocide. It has the great advantage of being a powder, easily soluble in water, and mailable to any part of the world. One teaspoonful in a pint of water makes a pleasant solution for wash, gargle, enema or for stomach administration.

A. E. Webber, 154 State Street, Springfield, Mass. Two ounces by mail, 50 cents.

PASTEURINE.

A strong germicide, a deodorant, non-irritating and pleasant to the nose and taste.

Belongs to the class embracing Listerine, Zymocide, etc., and may be substituted for them when more convenient.

Jno. T. Milliken & Co ,

St. Louis, Missouri.

PLATT'S CHLORIDES.

Henry B. Platt, 36 Platt Street, N. Y. Quart bottles, 50 cents.

An odorless, colorless, powerful disinfectant, of wide reputation, as it has been in use many years.

SANITAS DISINFECTING CANDLES.

American & Continental Sanitas Company, 636 to 642 West 55th Street, New York city. Plain 20 cents, Watered Jacketed 25 cents.

Each candle contains one pound of sulphur, and is sufficient for the disinfection of from 1,000 to 1,200 cubic feet of air in a confined space. Much more convenient than the sulphur powder.

SODA, BI-CARBONATE OF.

A Russian surgeon claims that a two per cent. solution of bi-carbonate of soda, chemically pure, stops inflammation and the production of pus more rapidly than any other antiseptic.

SANITAS.

The American & Continental Sanitas Company, 636 to 642 West 55th Street, New York city.

Sanitas does not hide the foul smells of decomposition by an overpowering odor of its own, but it generates oxygen in its most active form, and destroys all offensive matter and disease germs, and is free from the dangers attending the use of the poisonous metallic salts employed as disinfectants. A powerful air purifier, but not a consumer of oxygen. It is prepared by oxidizing the essential oils of the pine and the eucalyptus.

Where contagious diseases exist, Sanitas may be used freely. For ordinary purposes, Sanitas fluid is the best. The powder may be used in the same way as other disinfecting powders.

ZYMOCIDE.

Reed & Carnrick, Manufacturing Chemists, New York. Eight ounces 75 cents; fourteen ounces $1.

Cleansing, healing, colorless, non-poisonous, non-irritating liquid antiseptic. Will not stain or injure the most delicate fabric. A deodorizer in all suppurative and offensive discharges. Applied as a spray, douche or gargle. As an anti-ferment in cholera infantum, summer complaint, typhoid fever and digestive disorders.

One of the most elegant preparations ever offered.

The mistake should not be made of substituting a deodorizer for a disinfectant. An odor may be masked without the destruction of the attendant disease germs. The germs themselves may have no odor, therefore the danger may be just as great when the sense of smell detects nothing amiss, as when it is almost suffocated with effluvia.

Other disinfectants are here named in the order of their strength, but the weaker should not be relied upon in serious diseases.

Corrosive sublimate, 64 grains to the gallon.

Carbolic acid, 5 per cent. solution.

Bromine, 1 pound to 200 gallons.

Permanganate of potash, $17\frac{3}{4}$ ounces to 200 gallons.

Chloride of lime, 4 ounces to the gallon.

Sulphate of iron, $1\frac{1}{2}$ pounds to the gallon.

Sulphate of zinc, 4 ounces to the gallon.

Common salt, 2 ounces to the gallon.

STIMULANTS.

Stimulants are substances that arouse vital action. That they have a place in the physical economy is evident from the impossibility of distinguishing the dividing line between the effect of proper foods and that of weak stimulants.

It might also be inferred from the fact that man is constituted not only to act in response to, but to develop intellectual strength by mental stimulants.

It might also be argued from the fact that men instinctively resort to stimulants in certain conditions, as do animals likewise.

But this can never justify the use of intoxicating drinks as a beverage, nor the habitual table use of condiments.

The physiological effect of stimulants is to increase the red-blood cells for a few days, but unless fresh material for them to live upon is also supplied they soon perish, proving conclusively that the normal use for stimulation is transient only.

The weakness of the idea of toning the system by so-called tonics is just here.

Their tonicity consists in their power of stimulation. But as the system loses its susceptibility to feel that stimulation with every repetition of the dose, and as the drug gives no nutriment to the cells first proliferated, it follows that no really tonic effect is possible.

What seems such in some cases is the first effect of stimulation supported and made permanent by added nutrition.

There is a class of extreme cases in which the ordinary effects of stimulation are overborne and benefit secured, e. g., whiskey by the pint for snake bites, in which the alcohol acts as a germicide ; brandy or whiskey, a pint or more in twenty-four hours, in some cases of double pneumonia, etc., in which the alcohol acts as a force food and as a germicide, and its stimulation supports (temporarily) the vital energies.

But as a rule—

It is only when the vital powers need to be aroused temporarily that their use should be permitted.

Capsicum, or red pepper, is a pure stimulant, by far the best and safest for use under nearly all circumstances, and is a powerful antiseptic.

Mustard, externally, comes next ; and there is scarcely any form of depression that cannot be more safely and successfully met by one or both of these than by any drug or drugs of the materia medica.

The capsicum may be used in from one to three-grain doses, repeated according to the urgency of the symptoms from one to six hours.

The mustard, in the form of plasters, dry rubs, or in baths deserves far more general use than it has, *c. g.*, in the determination of blood to a part, the application of a mustard plaster to its immediate vicinity, and as soon as the surface reddens thoroughly, that removed and another just beyond its further border, and so on, until an extremity is reached, will often remove the most stubborn cases of congestion.

RELAXANTS.

Relaxants are substances that loosen the texture of the fibres of the tissues, and are useful in rigid conditions. The warm bath is one of the best. Ladies' slipper and lobelia are the best herbal relaxants.

Lobelia is decried by Allopaths because, they claim, that in two or three instances in the history of medicine it has had a fatal effect, but there is no positive proof of a single instance, while there is positive proof of fatal results in thousands of cases from drugs that they prescribe freely every day, *e. g.*, who does not know that morphine has slain its thousands. Morphine is a relaxant, but the further its effects extend the more disturbed do the pulsations become. On the other hand, the more pronounced the effect of lobelia, *the more regular does the pulse become.*

ASTRINGENTS.

Astringents are substances that contract and tighten the fibres of the tissues, consequently relaxants and astringents are exact opposites. That their use is admissable to some extent, may be inferred from the fact that both exist in foods that are instinctively sought, e. g., some fruits are strongly astringent while others are relaxant.

It often happens that one or the other of these, used for its appropriate condition, is a great reinforcement to the Cell-Salts, and even to the germicidal remedies that may be required. Among the most available and harmless astringents are blackberry roots, oak bark, geranium, hemlock bark, tanic acid, witch hazel, sumac and cinnamon.

Tonics only differ from astringents in that they are supposed to have a more permanent impression. The wisdom of their use is very questionable.

CHAPTER VII.

THE INDEPENDENT AND THE CO-OPERATIVE CURATIVES OF CHRISTIAN FAITH.

This book was first announced to the public as in course of preparation in June, 1896, but for various reasons was not given to the printer until June 7, 1897.

Notwithstanding present haste to issue it, I cannot allow it to close without a brief final chapter upon "The Independent and The Co-operative Curatives of Christian Faith."

The best statement of *The Independent Curative* is found in James 5:13–15:

> "Is any sick among you? let him call for the elders of the church; and let them pray over him. anointing him with oil in the name of the Lord: and the prayer of faith shall save the sick, and the Lord shall raise him up."

The *doctrine* is simply this:

The prayer of faith shall save the sick. But inasmuch as we "know not what to pray for as we ought," i. e., whether it is our privilege to pray in faith for recovery, God informs us by a certain process explained in Romans 8:26: "The Spirit itself maketh intercession for us with groanings (sighings) which cannot be uttered." That is, the Holy Spirit within us helps our pleadings, impels to vehement wrestlings for the desired good, and whenever that Spirit-helped intercession is felt, it is God's personal assurance that it *is* "according to His will" (verse 27) that this boon shall be granted upon the one condition of the faith of the supplicant.

That this doctrine produces accordant FACTS I KNOW
by more than one personal experience, but notably by the
healing of my lameness of twenty-five years' standing, as
narrated in—

"MY TWENTY-FIFTH YEAR JUBILEE,"

published in 1875.

That it was made the subject of ridicule by many is true ;
but I wish to write in this. my latest work, that, while
there are some slight matters in that narrative that probably would not have been stated in just the words they were
had they been written some years later, *yet no* FACT *was
misstated;* and after twenty years of experience, and much
investigation of the physical, psychical and religious principles involved, I KNOW, as well as I know the fact of
my conversion, that my cure was an act of Divine healing,
independent of the use of natural remedial agents.

Furthermore, I am positively certain, that the same principles and methods of reasoning by which it was sought to
be explained upon natural principles, if applied to personal religious experience, would unchristianize every
Christian who now lives or ever has lived, if accepted.

Note the doctrine well—its limitations and its safeguard.
God's will is the arbiter. That will—disclosed by the
Holy Spirit in the heart of the sufferer—is the personal
encouragement to the act of faith.

It is useless to inquire *why* He selects one, and passes
by the multitude. I only know that it is *not* because of
the superior piety, talents or influence of the chosen ones ;
but the positive elements that determine His choice must
remain unknown in this life.

The practical application of the subject in a domestic
medical work is simply this, viz. : It is right for the sufferer to offer the *testing* prayer to see if it receives the in-

tercessional help, without which the prayer for cure should be changed to a prayer that the affliction may be sanctified to the soul's good, and blessed to the good of others; but *with* which—

> "To doubt would be di-loyalty,
> To falter would be sin."

King Asa "in his disease sought not the Lord, but to the physicians." "And Asa slept with his fathers "—2 Chron. 16·12-13.

THE CO-OPERATIVE HELPS OF CHRISTIAN FAITH involve the same principles of God's sovereign will offering the privilege, and man's faith personally and consciously claiming it, but instead of receiving the help without the intervention of naturally curative agents, it is expected through such means. Sometimes with no specially suggested ones; at other times with the means clearly defined and imperative. In either case there is a curative efficiency displayed far beyond the mere encouragement of expectancy of relief, yet, may be, quite indefinite in measure, or may include complete recovery.

The Christian should never fail to seek this help. Its workings are amid the primal movements of cell-formation just where life lays its hand upon insensate matter, and bids it to live. Hence, its help is radical.

But the seeking should always be in the same spirit in which His independent help is sought—not with resignation, for there is no room for resignation unless the petition is denied—but with a spirit of consecrated subjection that will at once become resignation upon occasion.

"In those days was Hezekiah sick unto death. . . . Then he turned his face to the wall and prayed." . . . And Isaiah was sent to him with this message· "I have heard thy prayer, and have seen thy tears; behold, I will heal thee." . . . "And Isaiah said, take a lump of figs. And they took and laid it on the boil, (probably malignant carbuncle), and he recovered." 2 Kings. 20·1, 2, 5, 7.

THE
BIOCHEMIC CELL-SALTS.
3=GRAIN 6X TABLETS;

The same as used by Dr. S. H. Platt the last four years, and furnished
by him to his patients and patrons to the extent of
millions of doses.

THE PRESCRIPTIONS IN
"HOME TREATMENT WITH CELL-SALTS"

Were written with special reference to these 3-grain, 6x Salts

Six-x is the potency preferred in general practice by Dr. Schuessler, the
founder of the Biochemic System.

100 Doses any Cell=Salt Glass Bottle, 40 Cents, Post-paid.

**1200 Doses, Selected by Customer, in Glass Bottles, Pre-
paid, $4.**

E. F. BARNES,
Lock Box 24, Southern Pines, N. C.

Canada Agency, F. B Wells, Revelstoke, B C.

New England Agency, J S. Thompson, Goffstown, N. H

Western Agencies, see FOODS AND HELPS.

346

347

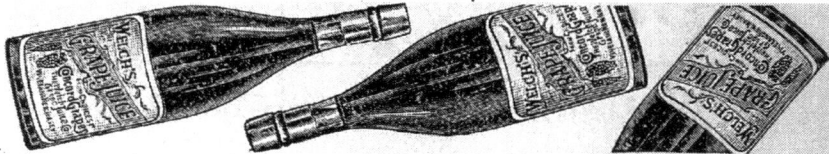

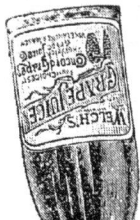

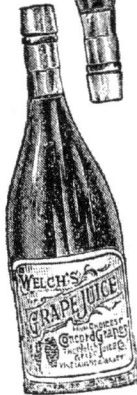

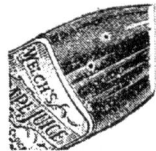

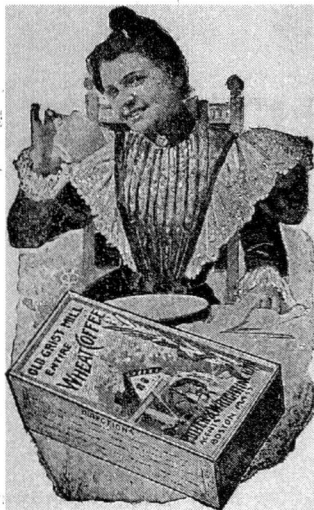

349

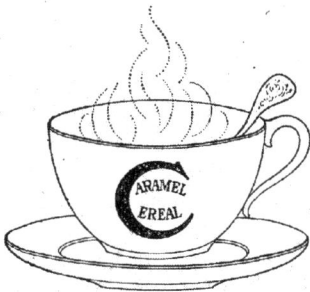

INDEX--GLOSSARY.

A

rumbling in, 96; torpor of, 100; ulceration, 134; wind (flatus) in 99–100.

Brain, 203–204; congestion of, 147; fag, 266; pains in, 224.

Bread, entire wheat recipe, 283.

Breathing, 192–194.

Breast, knots in, 133; tumors in, 133.

Bright's Disease, 136.

Bronchi, the two main branches of the windpipe, 194.

Bronchial Tubes and Throat, 192.

Bronchitis, inflammation of bronchi, 146; clinical cases, 21.

Bromo Chloralum, 333.

Bromose, 280.

Bromine, 333.

Bruises, 127.

Bunion, 127.

Burns and Scalds, 115.

C

Cachexia, constitutional drift to a certain disease, 21.

Calory, the amount of heat that will raise one pound of water 4° F. The number of calories that food generates is of great importance. If deficient the animal heat cannot be maintained; if excessive it tends to produce inflammations and fevers, 276.

Calc. Phos., chief characteristics, 68; functions of, 67.

Calc. Sulph., chief characteristics, 69; functions of, 68.

Calc. Fluor., chief characteristics, 70; functions of, 69.

Calves, sensations in, 252.

Camping-out parties, 312–313.

Cancer, 127; of stomach, C. Case, 21.

Canker, 128.

Capillary, hair-like; capillaries, the small tubes between the arteries and veins, 299, 300

Carbon, an elementary combustible substance, not metallic in nature, which predominates in all organic compounds and forms the base of charcoal and mineral coals, 69.

Carbohydrates, starches and sugar with exactly enough oxygen to saturate the hydrogen. Most convenient, 279; work of, 275; chemical, symbol of, C. H. O., 276.

Carbuncles, 128; infiltration of tissues after, 131. C. case, 22.

Carriage-riding, 305.

Casein (Protein), the alkali albumen of milk, 288

Cases, clinical, cases in their own practice reported by physicians to physicians, 18–61.

Cathartic, a drug that causes free movement of the bowels, 67.

Catarrh, 106–110; of stomach C. case, 23.

Catarrhal, affections, 153.

Catarrhal, inflammation, 108–109.

Cataract, 128.

Cautery, 319.

Cell-Salts, compensative functions of, 77; dosage, 87; efficiency of, 16; externally, 88; how they cure disease, 78; how to select, 273; higher potencies of, 85; normally existing in 3½ ounces of blood cells, 84; overdosed or misapplied, 14; preparation of, 80; properties and functions of, 66; relative waste of, 84; standard potency, 17; tablets, one or three grain, 88; trituration of, 80; what they are, 65–66; why deficient, 63; waste in twenty-four hours, 84.

Cell Evolution, 67.

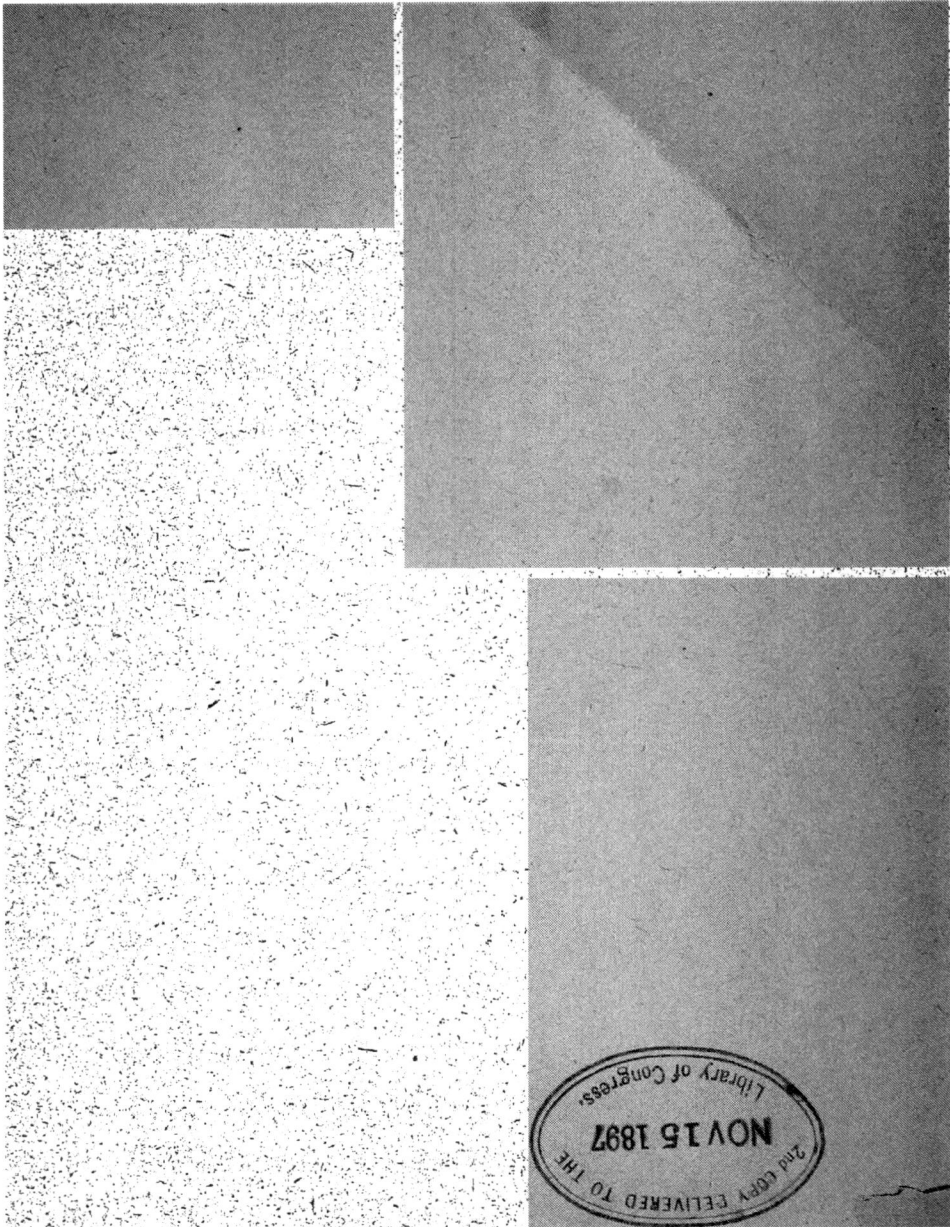

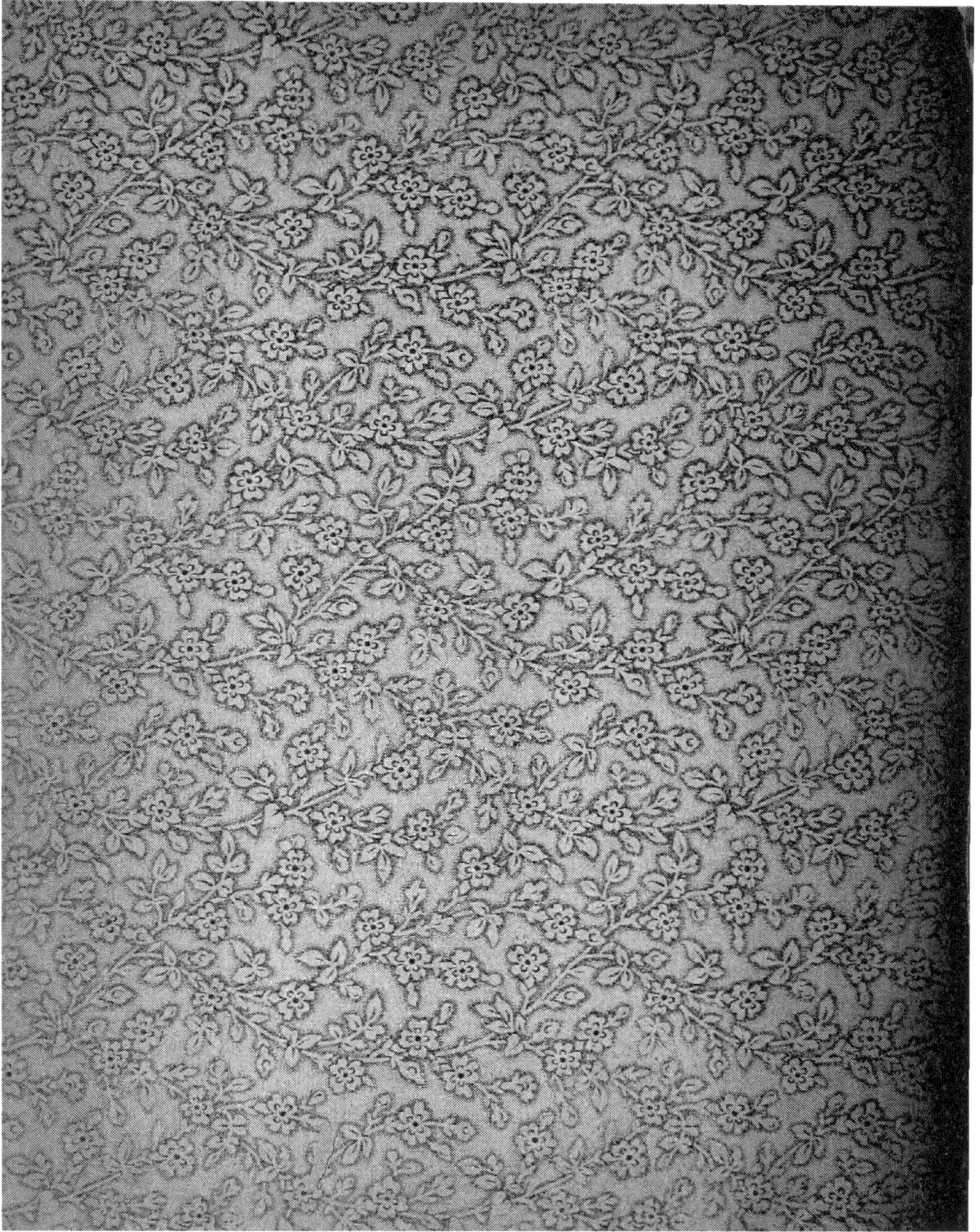

Milton Keynes UK
Ingram Content Group UK Ltd.
UKHW022020010124
435322UK00005B/247

9 781017 859058